Keto vegetarian cookbook

Try 300 different recipes to stay lean all year round.21 days meal plan included

Table of Contents

Introduction

If you already have an inbred fear for fatty foods or you are going to have a problem cutting down on your carb intake, then you may find it quite challenging to engage in keto. The ketogenic diet which basically implies limiting your daily dosage of carbohydrates and increasing your fat intake can actually be tough to start, especially for people who find it hard to transit from on diet to another.

The fear is normal since it involves a radical switch from your normal way of eating (The typical America standard diet involves a lot of carbohydrates and processed foods). However, the fears can be unfounded sometimes as the keto diet has little or no side effects for beginners, apart from the keto flu which has already been discussed in this book, and which can also be managed effectively. Relatively, the benefits that accrue to the keto diet are numerous and since a lot of people are engaging in it, including celebrities alike, then there is nothing stopping you from giving it a try.

As substantiated already, the main reason for the adoption of the keto diet is to drag the body into a stage called ketosis. Ketosis is what happens when the body turns from burning carbs for its daily energy need to expending fats as its main source of energy. Ketosis is necessary as it has been linked with fat burning and weight loss and so far, it has proved an effective way of dealing with those two nagging problems as well as other health related issues.

The big question now is; how do you prepare yourself for a journey into the keto diet? let us take a look at a few tips that will ease you into this diet without having to stress yourself.

1. Know What Foods You'll Eat and Avoid on the Ketogenic Diet

Following a keto diet mean plan and food list will have you cutting down severely on your carb intake. It is recommended that you start off with consuming somewhere between 20 to 30 grams of carbs on a daily basis.

You should also ensure that you are in the know about what food to eat, which of them is prevalent in carbohydrates and which has the right amount of fat required. This will enable you make the right choices about what to eat and what not to eat. For example, you should know that it's not just candy, chips, pasta, cookies, ice cream and bread that contains carbs, you can also find a defined amount of carb in beans even though they are classified under protein. Fruits and some veggies are also high carbs. The only foods that don't contain carbs are meat and pure fats which include the likes of butter and oils. Some of the oils can include olive oil and coconut oil.

2. Examine Your Relationship with Fat — Keto Involves Lots of It!

A lot of people are afraid of fat because of the notion that it can kill them. In order to get yourself ready for a high fat diet, which can be quite uncomfortable for some people at first, you have to begin with making small adjustments to what you eat daily. For instance, you can choose to order for burger on lettuce leaves while picking green veggies as alternatives for fries.

Instead of incorporating rice or potatoes into your meal plan, go for non-starchy veggies. Introduce more oil to your daily cooking. You should also be aware of the fact that your old dieting habits, like preparing a plain skinless grilled chicken breast is never compatible with keto diet because you stand the risk of not getting enough fat.

Start slowly with the process of substituting your carbs with fat. If you are afraid of fat, then be rest assured that the keto diet won't work for you.

3. Improve On Your Cooking Skills for A Fresh Start, As High Carb Processed Foods Should Never Make Its Way to Your Keto Meal Plan

You can improve on your cooking skills by taking a look at websites with keto friendly recipes as well as keto cookbooks. You are sure to find keto recipes that you are going to love. You can go on a search for up to four or five recipes with foods that will catch your interest. This will ensure that you are not left standing with your hands in your pocket, wondering on what your next meal is going to look like.

4. Give Bulletproof Coffee a Try, It's One of the Recommended and Best Keto-Friendly Drinks

You can make your own delicious bulletproof coffee at your convenience by mixing butter and coconut oil with your coffee. This drink is designed to help you fight off constant hunger while ensuring that you have adequate time in your hands to plan out your next meal. However, you should also keep an eye out on how much coconut oil you consume as it has the potential of sending LDL or bad cholesterol levels soaring. If you are at an increased risk of battling heart disease as a result of family history or personal health issues, then you should consider skipping this drink, or better still, check in with your health practitioner for recommendations and advice.

5. Talk to Your Family About Your Weight Loss Goals on the Diet

Have a heart to heart talk with members of your family and make them understand your plans. They should be aware that you may have to start passing on the regular meal that they are used to, this will allow you prepare whatever you are to eat yourself and also make them know what your new habits are going to look like.

Also endeavor to assure them this is just a temporary adjustment as keto diets are only done on a short term basis, say three to six months. If, however, they raise their concerns on what you are about to do, reassure them with the fact that you have done your research and know exactly what you are going into. They may even have their own roles to play in your keto journey.

6. Know What Side Effects to Expect Like the Keto Flu for Example

For all the fantastic benefits that you get for engaging in keto diet (including weight loss), there is one big side effect that you are going to have to contend with, and that is the keto flu.

The keto flu is a term adopted for the period of commencement of keto dieting when your body tried to adjust to the new arrangement of having to burn fat and not carbs anymore for its source of fuel. While some people won't have any problem with this, a lot of others often have a miserable experience.

The symptoms are usually more defined within the first week or 10 days of starting with this mode of dieting. You may start to have a tough experience climbing staircases and an extreme feeling of lethargic in your limbs can't also be ruled off. You may also have to deal with a mental fog.

That is why it is recommended that you choose a date or week with less crazy schedules and obligations for starting off your keto journey. Choose a period when you can afford all the rest that you can. In the same veins, you should also consider toning down on your daily exercise within the first week or two in order to allow your body time to adjust to the new plan.

7. Increase Your Electrolytes as a Measure for Preventing or Mitigating Unpleasant Keto Side Effects

During the stage of ketosis, the kidney tends to excrete more electrolytes and water. You should ensure that you are getting the right amount of sodium and potassium required by the body to perform optimally. You can do this by incorporating more salt in your meals, eating non starchy vegetables and drinking salted bone broths.

8. Have an After Plan, Because Keto Isn't Meant to Be a Long-Term Weight Loss Solution

A keto diet is only meant to last for a short period of time, therefore, it is not a forever diet. While some people can adopt the use of keto a few times a year for specific reasons, others may engage in it as a one-time solution for weight loss or for a change in their eating habits.

Avoid rushing back to the standard American diet as you risk the chances of losing all that you have gained from adopting the keto diet including the risk of adding those weight that you have lost already. What should be topmost on your mind is how to shift your diet to something healthier which may include consuming less pasta, less sugar, less flour and less bread. You should also consider increasing the amount of veggies in your meal.

Chapter 1. How to get started with ketogenic vegetarian diet

Getting started isn't a feat as seemed and neither extremely easy that will make you abuse the benefits. I was skeptical about the diet when I learned about it after trying many other unsuccessful diets. However, the Keto diet has been such a blessing –else I wouldn't master the Keto art for three years and counting.

I compiled this list of five that I bet will push you into ketosis in the shortest possible time as your body pleases. Ready?

1. Settle The Score With Yourself

Starting a diet is not as easy as it may seem. Pushing yourself to eat foods that you are unused to isn't how our bodies were trained, especially after splurging on carbohydrates and regular sugars for so long.

Give yourself a me-to-me pep talk about your reasons, sacrifices, and goals for taking on the Keto diet and position yourself in a comfortable mental, financial, and lifestyle phase to help you start and ride on successfully.

2. Eat The Right Foods

As you know, the Keto macros are healthy fats, proteins, and carbohydrates at a percentage ratio of 80% or more of fats, 20% to 35% of proteins and 0% to 10% of carbohydrates.

It is essential to follow this rule as you pantry clean and grocery shop. Below, I share a list of foods to eat and not to eat, and recommend that you keep eating more according to the macro ratio to maintain ketosis.

3. Drink a Lot Of Water

I haven't heard of a thing as excessive water intake, which is as essential as any water sermon out there. As the body changes from dieting on high-carbs to high-fats, water plays an indispensable role in transporting nutrients well around the body while keeping you satiated for extended periods to reduce calorie intake from bad appetites.

4. Prepare For Keto Flu

I would have quitted my diet after the first four days had I not learned about the Keto flu before starting. The feeling of irritability, confusion, and a flu-like feeling was good enough to send me on sick leave.

Not to scare you; however, the Keto flu is just a sign that your body is responding to the new changes of feeding on high-carbs to feeding on high-fats. As the liver begins to break your fatty acids into ketones, you will experience symptoms like headaches, fatigue, irritability, confusion, etc. These are all right and can be managed by continuing with the diet, drinking a lot of water, and avoiding high-intensity activities.

5. Also, Take a Lot Of Rest

Sleep isn't for the weak, but for the serious, that needs to be in an excellent, healthy state.

Making sure to get regular eight hours of sleep and a few more hours during the day will keep you energized. Most notably, during your first two weeks of dieting, the body will need the extra energy when you feel easily fatigued.

It is often a common occurrence to find people who are often preoccupied with questions like, "What can a vegetarian eat?" The basic truth is that individuals who adopt the vegetarian lifestyle can actually eat whatever they want. The difference here is that people who decide to identify themselves with the vegetarian identity choose not to eat certain things by their own free will.

Just like everyone else, vegetarians have their reasons for sticking to a particular dietary lifestyle. Those reasons could span from health to love for animals or simply a distaste for meat. So if you happen to find yourself wondering the type of vegetarian that you want to be, then you have to take a look at what type of foods you want to avoid or actually include in your dietary lifestyle. You don't necessarily have to entirely fit into one of the following categories but it is necessary that you understand them as this is the first step towards setting your short term and long-term goals, if you eventually decide to stick to the vegan lifestyle. Here are the categories that will help you understand the different types of vegetarians that you are bound to meet.

1. Flexitarian or Semi-Vegetarian

This is one category that tries to tell you that you don't really have to be a vegetarian to be able to fall in love with vegetarian foods. Flexitarian which can be ascribed for the definition of someone who loves to explore with what they eat is a term that most describes semi vegetarians. These group people while attracted to consuming mostly vegetarian meals can occasionally eat meat at intervals.

2. Pescatarian

The term pescatarian is used to denote a set of vegetarians who abstain from eating virtually all animal flesh but engage in the consumption of fish. They can also be called pescatarian. Over time, more and more people are moving over to this particular category and this is usually based on health reasons or may serve as a starting point for those who have the desire to go fully vegetarian in the nearest feature. They use this stage as a selling stone.

3. Lacto-Ovo-Vegetarian

This is the mostly identified type of vegetarian diet known to most people everywhere. Usually, when the issue of vegetarian is raised, a lot of people will easily have their minds running towards lacto-ovo-vegerarians. These are a set of vegetarians who restricts themselves absolutely from the consumption of pork, beef, fish, poultry shellfish, or as a matter of fact, animal flesh of any kind. However, these set of people can also do with the consumption of eggs and other dairy products. The word "lacto" is coined from the Latin word for milk while "ovo" means egg. Lacto ovo vegetarians constitute a large amount of vegetarians and are the most commonly found across the world.

You can also choose to stick to one between egg or dairy products. A lacto-vegetarian defines a vegetarian who consumes dairy products but is restricted to eggs while ovo-vegetarian is used to refer to individuals who are restricted to meat and dairy products but consume eggs.

4. Vegan

Vegans are vegetarians that abstain from the consumption of all meat products of any kind. Included in this mix are eggs, dairy products or any processes food that has traces of these or other ingredients derives from animals such as gelatin which is extracted from animal collagen.

Some vegans are also known to shy away from the consumption of foods that are processed with animal products even though there are evidently no presence of such animal products in the finished food. For example, bone char is employed in the making of some sugars during the bleaching and filtering process while some wines are known to be processed with milk protein, egg whites and gelatin which serve as fining agents during the production stage, however, these products do not form the basic ingredients in the final output but then again, some vegans also try to avoid them. However, there are some debates citing the possibility of some foods like honey being fit to be classified as vegan diets.

5. Raw Vegan or Raw Food Diet

A raw vegan diet is made up of unprocessed vegan foods which must have not undergone a heating of above 115 F or 46 C. People who adopt this diet are referred to as raw foodist and this trend came to be as a result of the common belief that food heated above the stated temperature tend to lose a huge amount of their nutritional value and may turn out harmful for the body.

6. Macrobiotic

This diet, popular for its healthy and healing abilities is made up of unprocessed vegan foods including fruits, vegetables, whole grains and also allows for the consumption of fish at intervals. These set of vegetarian diets also restrict the consumption of sugar and refined oil.

Chapter 2. What to eat and What to avoid

FOODS TO EAT

You likely wonder how to bring this into exercise now that you understand what foods you need to be careful about on your vegetarian ketogenic diet. At first, it can look tricky to make vegetarian dishes. But you will build a collection of vegetarian recipes with a little researching and practice so that your diet is both nutritious and enjoyable.

Let us begin with listing some essential components that you must add to your refrigerator and cupboard:

Plant-based fats: Olives and its oils, avocados and its oil, coconut and its oil (but do not eat any sweetened coconut).

Low-carb vegetarian proteins: Seitan, tofu, and even tempeh; even if it is higher in carbs than tofu and seitan, it is also higher in fiber, which makes your net carbs keto-friendly. Be cautious about faux-meat burgers, bacon, etc. and check their list of ingredients and nutrition tags as they can contain sugar or as an unwanted carbs source.

Low-carb vegetables: Cauliflower of course, and also asparagus, swiss chard, brussels sprouts, cabbage, mushrooms, zucchini, broccoli rabe, spinach, bok choy, kale, and lettuces (romaine, arugula, green and red leaf, endive, and so on).

Nuts: When you eat vegetarian keto, every nut is the right choice, but some are higher in fat and lower in carbohydrates than the others, and these are pili nuts, macadamias, hazelnuts, and pecans.

Seeds: Here, you can't really go wrong. Seeds are fatty, not too high in carbohydrates and ordinarily full of fiber, which can cause your net carbs to fall.

Dairy: Hard cheeses, butter, full-fat plain yogurt, and plain cottage cheese (avoid the flavored high-sugar varieties).

Eggs: This is the easiest, healthiest, and most excellent way to get protein if you eat vegetarian keto. Eggs also give you a good dose of fat and almost no carbs.

Berries: Blackberries, strawberries, and raspberries all offer lower carb fruit choices. Not because they really have low carbohydrates, but because they have fiber and therefore your net carbohydrates are low. You may want to avoid blueberries because a cup will eat almost all of your daily carb allotment.

Condiments and spices: Soy sauce (light), apple cider vinegar (ACV), basil pesto, mayonnaise, mustard, hot sauce, ranch dressing, all spices, and herbs.

And, as valuable as it is to have a list of foods you can consume, you might also wish to list the foods you cannot eat (those foods that will throw you out of the status of ketosis), in order to successfully use a vegetarian ketogenic diet. These are legumes, cereals, most fruit and all kinds of potatoes.

While the keto diet cuts down on many food groups on which vegetarian depend, such as starchy vegetables and whole grains, cautious scheduling can be used to follow a vegetarian keto diet. Vegetarians should obtain their calories from whole and unprocessed foods while evading highly manufactured vegetarian meals.

FOODS TO AVOID

You should stay away from all meat and seafood in a vegetarian keto diet. High carbohydrates foods such as cereals, legumes, starchy vegetables, and fruit can only be allowed in tiny quantities, provided that they match your regular carb allotment.

The following foods have to be removed:

- Fish and shellfish: salmon, tuna, sardines, anchovies, and lobster

- Poultry: chicken, turkey, duck, and goose

- Meat: beef, pork, lamb, goat, and veal Here are certain foods you should restrict:

- Sweeteners: brown sugar, white sugar, honey, maple syrup, and agave nectar

- Sugar-sweetened beverages: soda, sweet tea, sports drinks, juice, and energy drinks

- Starchyvegetables:potatoes,yams, beets, parsnips, carrots, and sweet potatoes

- Fruits: apples, bananas, oranges, berries, melon, apricots, plums, and peaches

- Grains: bread, rice, quinoa, oats, millet, rye, barley, buckwheat, and pasta

- Processed foods: breakfast cereals, granola, chips, cookies, crackers, and baked goods

- Legumes: beans, peas, lentils, and chickpeas

- Condiments: barbecue sauce, honey mustard, ketchup, marinades, and sweetened salad dressings

- Alcoholic beverages: beer, wine, and sweetened cocktails

Chapter 3. Breakfast recipes

1. Cinnamon Flavored Blueberry Coffee Cake

Servings: 1 cake

Preparation Time: 30 min

Cooking Time: 75 min

Ingredients:

2 cups whole-wheat flour, sifted

1 teaspoon vanilla extract

1 ¼ cup honey, divided

¼ cup brown sugar, packed

1 ½ teaspoon ground cinnamon

¾ cup fat free yogurt

1 tablespoon baking powder

¼ teaspoon salt

½ cup soy milk, unsweetened

¾ cup butter, unsalted and soften

2 cup frozen blueberries, thawed

Directions:

Set oven at 350 degrees F and heat until cake is ready to bake.

Take a 9 inch round cake pan, grease with butter and set aside until required.

In a medium sized mixing bowl, place ¼ cup honey and brown sugar, and using a whisker stir in cinnamon until combined.

In another medium bowl, place 1 ¾ cups flour and using a whisker stir in baking powder and salt until just mixed.

In another medium size mixing bowl, whisk together milk and vanilla extract until combined.

In a large bowl, place ½ cup of butter and using an electric beater beat in remaining honey until creamy.

Beat in yogurt until smooth.

Gradually beat in flour mixture and milk-vanilla mixture, alternately, until moist and soft dough comes together.

Spoon half of the cake mixture into the prepared cake pan, drizzle with 2 tablespoons of cinnamon mixture and using skewer swirl the batter, and top with 1 cup of blueberries.

Spread remaining cake batter over the blueberries, drizzle with 2 tablespoons of cinnamon mixture and using skewer swirl the batter again, and top with 1 cup of blueberries.

Place a small saucepan over medium flame, heat remaining batter until melted, then using a whisker stir in remaining flour and cinnamon mixture and sprinkle over the cake.

Place cake pan in the heated oven and bake for 60-70 minutes until inserted wooden skewer into the center of cake comes out clean.

Let baked cake cool in the pan for 20 minutes on wire rack before turning out.

Slice to serve.

Nutrition:

467 Cal, 18 g total fat (5 g sat. fat), 0 mg chol., 468 mg sodium, 73 g carb., 2g fiber, 5 g protein, 42 g sugars.

2. Rosemary & Blueberry Scones

Servings: 6-8 scones

Preparation Time: 30 min

Cooking Time: 30 min

Ingredients:

2 ¼ whole-wheat flour, sifted

¾ cups milk, unsweetened

2 eggs

1 tablespoon baking powder

¼ cup maple syrup

½ teaspoon salt

1 tablespoon rosemary leaves, chopped

1/3 cup coconut oil, solid

¼ cups frozen blueberries, thawed

Directions:

Set oven at 400 degrees F and heat until scones are ready to bake.

Take a large baking tray, dust lightly with flour and set aside until required.

In a medium bowl, whisk together milk and 1 egg until combined and set aside until required.

In a food processor, place flour, baking powder, maple syrup, salt, rosemary and coconut oil, and pulse until mixture resembles breadcrumbs.

Tip the mixture into a large bowl, make a well in the center, pour in milk-egg mixture and using a spoon stir until soft and moist dough comes together.

If the dough is too dry, stir in 1-2 tablespoons almond milk and if the dough is too moist, stir in 1-2 tablespoons flour.

Fold in blueberries and transfer dough to a clean surface, dusted with flour.

Pat dough to flatten into 1 inch thick round.

Now dip a 2 ¼ inch scone cutter or biscuit cutter in the flour and cut out round scones by pressing directly down and lifting straightly up.

Combine the scraps of dough, pat into a round and cut out more scones.

Now line scones, side by side, on a prepared baking tray.

In a bowl, beat an egg and with a brush, coat the top of scones lightly.

Sprinkle sugar over the scones and place baking tray in the heated oven.

Bake scones for 25-30 minutes until golden brown and risen.

Cool baked scones on wire racks and then serve with butter and jam.

Nutrition:

334 Cal, 16.5 g total fat (13.2 g sat. fat), 0 mg chol., 431 mg sodium, 42.9 g carb., 3.4g fiber, 5.4 g protein.

3. Almond & Pomegranate Scones

Servings: 20 scones

Preparation Time: 30 min

Cooking Time: 20 min

Ingredients:

¾ cup whole-wheat flour, sifted

1 cup almond flour

3 tablespoons honey, and more as needed

¼ teaspoon salt

1 ½ teaspoons baking powder

1 egg

¼ cup almond milk

¼ teaspoon baking soda

3 tablespoons pomegranate juice, divided

4 tablespoons butter, unsalted and soften

½ cup frozen pomegranate, thawed

¼ cup confectioner's sugar

¼ cup sliced almonds

Directions:

Set oven at 400 degrees F and heat until scones are ready to bake.

Take a large baking tray, dust lightly with flour and set aside until required.

In a blender, place flour, baking soda, baking powder, honey, butter and pulse until mixture resembles grains.

Tip the flour mixture into a large bowl and set aside until required.

In another bowl, place 2 tablespoons pomegranate juice and using a whisker stir in milk until combined.

Gradually stir in milk mixture into flour mixture until soft and moist dough comes together.

If the dough is too dry, stir in 1-2 tablespoons almond milk and if the dough is too moist, stir in 1-2 tablespoons flour.

Fold in pomegranate seeds and transfer dough to a cleaned surface dusted with flour.

Pat dough to flatten into 1 inch thick rectangle.

Now dip a heart shaped scone cutter or biscuit cutter in the flour and cut out scones by pressing directly down and lifting straightly up.

Combine the scraps of dough, pat into a round and cut out more scones.

Now line scones, side by side, on prepared baking tray.

In a bowl, beat an egg and with a brush, coat the top of scones lightly.

Sprinkle sugar over the scones and place baking tray in the heated oven.

Bake scones for 15-20 minutes until golden brown and risen.

In the meantime, in a medium sized mixing bowl, place sugar and using a whisker stir in remaining 1 tablespoon pomegranate juice until combined.

Cool baked scones on wire racks, then drizzle with sugar-pomegranate mixture, sprinkle with almonds and serve.

Nutrition:

100 Cal, 6 g total fat (1 g sat. fat), 0 mg chol., 115 mg sodium, 11 g carb., 1g fiber, 2 g protein, 5 g sugars.

4. Sweet Potato Cornbread

Servings: 1 cornbread

Preparation Time: 30 min

Cooking Time: 30 min

Ingredients:

6 tablespoons butter, unsalted and soften

¾ cup whole-wheat flour

1 ¼ cup low fat buttermilk

1 2/3 cups cornmeal

1 tablespoon baking powder

1 teaspoon salt

2 eggs

2 cups sliced green collards

1 medium sweet potato, cooked and smashed

1/3 cup agave syrup

Directions:

Set oven at 375 degrees f and heat until cornbread is ready to bake.

Take a dark 9 by 2 inch baking pan; brush the inner sides generously with oil and set aside until required.

Place a medium non-stick skillet pan over low flame and heat 1 tablespoon butter until melted.

Add greens to the pan, season with salt, cover pan and cook for 5 minutes until softened, stir occasionally.

Transfer cooked collard greens to a plate and set aside until required.

In a medium sized mixing bowl, place flour and using a whisker stir in flour, agave syrup, salt and baking powder until just mixed.

In a separate large bowl, using an electric beater, cream remaining butter and then beat in mashed sweet potato, eggs and buttermilk until blended.

Fold in cooked collard greens and then stir in flour mixture, 2-3 tablespoons at a time, until soft and moist dough comes together.

If the dough is too moist, stir in 1-2 tablespoons flour and if the dough is too dry, stir in 1-2 tablespoons water.

Pour the batter into prepared baking pan, with spatula smooth top and place baking tray into heated oven.

Bake bread for 25-30 minutes until top is nicely golden brown and inserted wooden skewer into the center of bread comes out clean.

Cool bread in the pan for 10 minutes before turning out to cool completely. Slice to serve.

Nutrition:

201 Cal, 8 g total fat (4 g sat. fat), 48 mg chol., 383 mg sodium, 29 g carb., 4g fiber, 4 g protein, 8 g sugars.

5. Quinoa & Flax Muffins

Servings: 14 muffins

Preparation Time: 60 min

Cooking Time: 60 min

Ingredients:

¾ cup quinoa, uncooked

1 cup brown rice flour

¼ cup white rice flour

2 teaspoons baking soda

½ cup melted coconut oil

2 eggs

½ teaspoon salt

1/3 cup olive oil

2 ½ cup water

1 cup low fat buttermilk

¼ cup tapioca flour

3 tablespoons flaxseed

1 cup raisins

½ cup potato starch

1 teaspoon xantham gum

¼ teaspoon ground cinnamon

1 cup honey

1 cup chopped walnuts

Directions:

Place a large saucepan over medium high flame, place quinoa, pour in water and bring to boil, stir occasionally.

Then switch flame to medium and simmer for 20-30 minutes or until all the water is absorbed by quinoa, stir occasionally.

In the meantime, in a medium sized mixing bowl, place raisins, pour in enough boiling water to immerse the raisins and let stand for 30 minutes until plump.

When all the liquid is absorbed by quinoa, switch off the flame, fluff the mixture with a fork and transfer into a separate medium sized mixing bowl.

Add buttermilk and flaxseeds to the quinoa, stir until just mixed and let stand for 30 minutes.

Drain raisins and set aside until required.

Set oven at 375 degrees F and heat until pancakes are ready to bake.

Take a standard 14 cups dark muffin pan, having each cup of 2 ½ inches in diameter.

Line each cup with a paper liner and lightly drench with non-stick cooking spray or until just evenly coated, or dip a paper towel in oil and grease each cup generously, set aside until required.

In a separate medium sized bowl, sift together brown and white rice flour, potato starch, tapioca flour and stir in xantham gum, baking soda, salt and cinnamon until combined.

In a separate large bowl, using an electric beater beat eggs until frothy and then beat in honey and oil until creamy.

Stir in quinoa mixture and then gradually stir the mixture into flour mixture until soft and moist dough comes together.

Fold in raisins and walnuts and using an ice cream scoop, divide the muffin batter evenly among prepared muffin cups.

Place muffin pan in the heated oven and bake muffins for 25 to 30 minutes until muffins expand, the rounded top brown nicely and inserted wooden skewer into center of muffins comes out clean.

Cool muffin pan on wire rack for 10 minutes before turning out and then serve warm.

Nutrition:

268 Cal, 7 g total fat (1 g sat. fat), 27 mg chol., 483 mg sodium, 49 g carb., 2g fiber, 5 g protein, 25 g sugars.

6. Corn Muffins

Servings: 6-8 muffins

Preparation Time: 5 min

Cooking Time: 20 min

Ingredients:

1 egg

1 cup cornmeal

½ cup whole-wheat flour, sifted

2 teaspoons baking powder

 2 tablespoons coconut sugar

2 tablespoons melted coconut oil

1 cup water

½ teaspoon salt

Directions:

Set oven at 450 degrees F and heat until pancakes are ready to bake.

Take a standard 6 cups dark muffin pan, having each cup of 2 ½ inches in diameter.

Line each cup with a paper liner and lightly drench with non-stick cooking spray or until just evenly coated, or dip a paper towel in oil and grease each cup generously, set aside until required.

In a large bowl, using an electric beater beat egg until foamy and then beat in oil and water until blended.

In a medium bowl, place cornmeal and using a whisker stir in flour, baking powder, coconut sugar and salt until just mixed.

Stir flour mixture into egg mixture 2-3 tablespoons at a time until soft and moist dough comes together.

If the dough is too hard, stir in 1-2 tablespoons water and if the dough is too moist, stir in 1-2 tablespoons flour.

Using an ice cream scoop, divide the muffin batter evenly among prepared muffin cups and place pan in the heated oven.

Bake muffins for 20-25 minutes until muffins expand, the rounded top brown nicely and inserted wooden skewer into center of muffins comes out clean.

Cool muffin pan on wire rack for 10 minutes before turning out and then serve warm.

Nutrition:

199 Cal, 4g total fat (2 g sat. fat), 0 mg chol., 202 mg sodium, 37 g carb., 2g fiber, 3 g protein.

7. Cranberry & Almond Biscotti

Servings: 20-22 cookies

Preparation Time: 30 min

Cooking Time: 60 min

Ingredients:

1 ¼ cups whole-wheat flour, sifted

1 teaspoon baking powder

1/8 teaspoon salt

6 ½ tablespoons orange juice

2 tablespoons cornstarch

½ cup honey

2 tablespoons brown sugar

1 tablespoon melted coconut oil

½ teaspoon almond extract

½ teaspoon vanilla extract

½ cup dried cranberries

½ cup sliced almonds

Directions:

Place baking rack in the middle of oven, set temperature at 350 degrees F and heat until biscotti are ready to bake.

In the meantime, take two large flat baking trays, line with baking paper and set aside until required.

In a large bowl, place flour, baking powder, salt and stir until just mixed.

In a small bowl, place 2 ½ tablespoons orange juice and cornstarch together and set aside until required.

In a separate large mixing bowl, place ½ cup honey and using an electric beater beat in remaining orange juice, oil, vanilla and almond extracts until fluffy.

Then beat in cornstarch mixture until smooth.

Stir in flour mixture, 2-3 tablespoons at a time, until soft dough comes together.

Add cranberries and almonds to the batter and fold until just mixed.

Using an ice cream scoop, arrange dough portions, at least 5-8, in rows on the lined baking trays, at some distance between them.

Use spatula to press down for flattening each dough portion slightly and then chill in refrigerator for 20 minutes.

Brush milk on surface of biscuits, sprinkle with sugar and bake in the heated oven for 40-45 minutes until nicely golden brown.

Let baked biscuits stand in baking tray for 5 minutes before dividing by running knife diagonally through each biscuit.

Bake biscuits again for 15-20 minutes until brown and cool completely on wire rack before serving.

Nutrition:

82 Cal, 2 g total fat, 0 mg chol., 38 mg sodium, 15 g carb., 1g fiber, 1 g protein.

8. Onion Stuffed Flatbread

Servings: 8

Preparation Time: 20 min

Cooking Time: 15 min

Ingredients:

2 cups whole-wheat flour, sifted

½ teaspoon salt

3 tablespoons olive oil, and more as needed

3 medium onions

1 teaspoon ground coriander

1 teaspoon chopped jalapeno pepper

1 teaspoon lemon juice

Directions:

In a food processor, place flour, salt and olive oil, and pulse until mixture resembles breadcrumbs.

Tip the mixture in a large bowl, gradually mix 1 ¼ cups water until soft dough comes together.

Cover the bowl with a kitchen cloth and let dough rest in a warm place for 10 minutes.

In the meantime, chop onions and place in a bowl. Add coriander, jalapeno and lemon juice and stir until just combined.

After 10 minutes, uncover dough, place a clean working space dusted with flour and divide into 8 equal portions and roll into balls.

Dust flour over dough balls and using rolling pin, roll each ball into 3 inches diameter circle.

Place a heaping spoon of onion filling in the center of each circle, seal by joining the dough edges together and crimp tightly.

Place balls crimped side down, dust with flour and using rolling pin, roll each piece into 6 inches circle.

Place a large non-stick skillet over medium flame and let heat. Cook bread, one at a time, for 1 minutes until bottom starts golden brown and firm.

Brush the top of bread with oil, flip and cook for another 2 minutes until the other side is nicely brown and firm, press bread to cook evenly.

Brush the top of bread with oil, flip and cook for 1-2 minutes until the opposite side of bread is evenly brown, press bread to cook evenly.

Cook remaining breads in the same manner and serve hot.

Nutrition:

192 Cal, 5 g total fat (8 g sat. fat), 0 mg chol., 148 mg sodium, 29 g carb., 3g fiber, 5 g protein.

9. Eggless Garlic Bread Rolls

Servings: 3

Preparation Time: 130 min

Cooking Time: 45 min

Ingredients:

1 ½ cups whole-wheat flour, sifted

2 tablespoons all-purpose flour, sifted

1 teaspoon instant yeast, dry

2/3 cups warm water

¾ tablespoon coconut sugar

1 ½ tablespoons olive oil, divided

½ teaspoon salt

2 tablespoon butter, fat free

¾ tablespoon minced garlic

1 teaspoon chopped celery

¼ teaspoon oregano

1/8 teaspoon carom seeds

¾ teaspoon salt

Ground black pepper - ¼ tsp

Sesame seeds, as needed

Directions:

In a large bowl, place yeast, water and sugar, stir once and let yeast sit for 12-15 minutes in a warm place until foamy.

In the meantime, in a food processor, place flours, salt and 1 tablespoon oil, and pulse for 2 minutes until mixture resemble breadcrumbs.

Tip the mixture into frothy yeast mixture and mix well.

Then using hands, knead mixture for 3-5 minutes until soft and smooth dough comes together.

Brush dough with oil, cover with kitchen towel and let dough rest in a warm place for 1 to1 ½ hours until dough doubles in size.

In the meantime, place butter in a medium size bowl and using electric beater beat until creamy. Then beat in garlic, celery, oregano, carom seeds, salt, black pepper and remaining oil until combined.

Transfer raised dough onto a clean working space dusted with flour, punch lightly and divide into two equal portions.

Using rolling pin, roll one portion of dough into a circle of ½ inch thickness, and spread with prepared creamy garlic mixture.

Starting with one side of the dough, roll to the other end.

Make similar roll of the other portion of the dough.

Now, using a sharp knife make a cut at the center of each roll and then make another cut at the center of each roll, making eight rolls.

Take a large skillet pan and grease with oil generously and place eight rolls.

Brush remaining creamy garlic mixture on the top of rolls, sprinkle with sesame seeds, cover the pan and let rolls rest for 35-45 minutes until double in size.

In the meantime, place baking rack in the middle of the oven, set temperature at 3-5 degrees F and heat until rolls are ready to bake.

Place pan in the heated oven and bake for 35-45 minutes until top of rolls is nicely golden brown and rolls are firm.

Serve warm.

Nutrition:

94 Cal, 2.04 g total fat (0.48 g sat. fat), 0 mg chol., 145 mg sodium, 14 g carb., 3g fiber, 2.35 g protein.

10. Broccoli & Tofu Stuffed Pita Pockets

Preparation Time: 60 min

Cooking Time: 50 min

Ingredients:

1 ½ cups whole-wheat flour

1 cup all-purpose flour

½ teaspoon instant yeast, dry

1 ¼ warm water

½ teaspoon salt

1 medium broccoli head

12 ounce tofu, extra firm

2 tablespoons minced garlic

2 teaspoons olive oil, divided

1 medium onion

1 tablespoon ground coriander

1 teaspoon ground cumin

1 teaspoon hot chili pepper

¾ teaspoon salt, and more as needed

¾ cup chopped spinach

¾ cup chopped Kale

1 teaspoon mustard seeds

1 teaspoon red pepper flakes

Directions:

In a large bowl, place yeast, water and sugar, stir once and let yeast sit for 12-15 minutes in a warm place until foamy.

Into frothy yeast mixture, add flours and using hands mix and knead for 3-5 minutes until soft and smooth dough comes together.

Brush dough with oil, cover bowl with kitchen towel and let dough rest in a warm place for 1 - 1 ½ hours until dough doubles in size.

Transfer raised dough onto a clean working space dusted with flour, punch down and divide the dough into 1 inch diameter balls.

In the meantime, roughly chop broccoli, add to a food processor and pulse until shredded.

Roll dough parts into smooth balls, cover with kitchen towel and let them stand for 10 minutes.

In the meantime, place a medium non-stick skillet over medium flame and heat 1 tablespoon oil until hot.

Mince onion in a food processor, add to pan and cook for 5-8 minutes until translucent.

Add garlic to the pan and cook for 1 minute.

Stir in coriander, cumin, chili until well mixed.

Add broccoli, season with salt and cook for 7-10 minutes until tender and all the moisture in the pan evaporate, stir frequently.

While the broccoli is cooking, rinse tofu under running water, crumble and then add to the cooked broccoli.

Adjust the salt and cook until all the moisture in the pan evaporate. Set aside broccoli mixture and let cool.

Place baking rack in the middle of oven, set oven at 450 degrees F and let heat until calzones are ready to bake.

Place a medium non-stick frying pan over medium low flame and heat remaining 1 tablespoon oil until hot.

Add mustard seeds and cook until they start to sputter.

Then add red pepper flakes, spinach and kale, season with 1 teaspoon salt and stir until just mix.

Cover pan and let vegetables cook until tender.

Adjust salt in the vegetables, set aside the pan and let vegetables cool.

Work on the dough balls. Using rolling pin Roll each dough ball into 4-5 inch diameter circle or until thin.

Working on one circle at a time, place 3 tablespoons of broccoli-tofu filling in the center of each circle and top with cooked greens.

Brush the edges of circle with water and fold one half of the circle over the other, forming semicircle.

Seal the semicircle by pressing the edges and crimping using a fork.

Prepare remaining semicircles in the same manner and place on a large baking sheet, greased with oil.

Brush calzones (semicircleswith oil and place in the oven to bake for 15-20 minutes until nicely golden brown and crispy.

Let calzones cool on wire racks doe 10 minutes before serving with condiment.

Nutrition:

317 Cal, 21 g total fat (11 g sat. fat), 143 mg chol., 392 mg sodium, 21 g carb., 1g fiber, 11 g protein.

11. Blueberry Oatmeal Waffles

Servings: 6 waffles

Ingredients:

1 cup white whole wheat flour, sifted

1 teaspoon baking powder

½ teaspoon salt

¼ teaspoon ground allspice

1 cup quick oats

1/3 cup unsweetened applesauce

1 ½ cup reduced fat milk

2 tablespoons olive oil

1 teaspoon vanilla extract

1 ½ cups fresh blueberries

Directions:

In a large mixing bowl, place flour and using a whisker stir in allspice, oats, baking powder and salt until just mixed.

Make a well in the center of bowl, and pour in oil, vanilla, milk, maple syrup and mix until moist dough comes together and then let rest for 5 minutes.

If the batter is too thick, stir in 1-2 tablespoons water, and if the batter is too moist, stir in 1-2 tablespoons wheat flour.

In the meantime, switch on the waffle iron, grease with oil generously and heat.

Add blueberries into waffle mixture, stir until just mix and then pour batter into waffle iron, enough that the waffle iron is not overfilled and neither the outer edges of the iron.

Cook waffle until crispy and reach to desire color.

Prepare remaining waffles in the same manner.

Let waffles cool before serving with maple syrup.

Nutrition:

93.7 Cal, 10.1 g total fat (2 g sat. fat), 45 mg chol., 304 mg sodium, 26.8 g carb., 1.5g fiber, 6.2 g protein.

12. Breakfast Pudding - Apple Crumble

This breaking pudding with oats and apple energizes you. Top with nuts, dried fruit for a crunchy effect.

Servings: 6

Preparation Time: 10 Minutes

Cooking Time: 4 hrs. on LOW or 2 hrs. on HIGH

 Ingredients

Pudding:

1 cup - unsweetened milk (or use unsweetened almond milk)

2 cups - water

2 tbsps. - maple syrup

½ cup - chia seeds

2 tbsps. - arrowroot powder (or corn starch)

1 tsp - cinnamon (ground)

A pinch - rock salt

5 large - apples with skin, (sliced)

Cinnamon Crunch Topping:

½ cup - blanched almond flour

¼ cup - shredded coconut

¼ cup - coconut sugar (or use honey)

1 tsp - cinnamon

¼ cup - apple sauce (unsweetened)

1 tsp -pure vanilla extract

Directions:

Mix water, milk, maple syrup, chia seeds, arrowroot or cornstarch, salt and cinnamon to crockpot.

Place the sliced apples on top

Mix ingredients for crumble topping in a bowl. Spread this over the apples.

Cook on LOW heat for 4 hours or on HIGH heat for 2 hours.

Cool for an hour. Serve with dried fruit and nuts

13. Pumpkin Granola

Servings: 6

Preparation Time: 10 Minutes

Cooking Time: 4 hrs.

 Ingredients

2 1/2 cups - rolled oats (or gluten free oats)

8 tbsp. - pumpkin puree (canned)

1/2 - cup honey

1/2 cup - whole almonds (or toasted pumpkin seeds)

1/2 cup - dried cranberries or raisins (any dried fruit mixture)

1/2 tbsp. - pumpkin pie spice

1/2 tsp - cinnamon (ground)

1/2 tsp - kosher salt

Directions:

Add all ingredients except the dried fruit. Cover and cook on HIGH for 4 hours. Stir the mixture every 30 minutes.

Add dried fruit in the last hour of cooking. Let it cool for a while.

Serve once cooled or store in fridge for later.

14. 3-Grain Porridge

Servings: 8

Preparation Time: 10 Minutes

Cooking Time: 4 1/2 - 5 hrs.

 Ingredients

1/2 cup - millet

1/2 cup - buckwheat

1/2 cup - amaranth grains

2 - Large apples (peeled and chopped)

1 tsp – cinnamon

1/2 tsp – allspice

1/4 tsp – ginger

1/8 tsp – cardamom

1/2 tsp – salt

1 tsp – vanilla

1/4 cup - raw coconut sugar (or honey)

1/4 cup - molasses (optional)

5 1/2 cups – water

Almonds or walnuts to garnish

Directions:

Mix all ingredients in pot. Cover with lid and cook on LOW for 4 1/2 to 5 hours. Cook it for longer if you want a thicker consistency.

Top with almonds or walnuts and serve with milk.

15. Grits

Servings: 6-7servings

Preparation Time: 10 Minutes

Cooking Time: 6-8 hrs.

 Ingredients

1 cup - grits

5 cups - water

1/4 cup - butter

1/2 tsp - kosher salt

Shredded cheese as topping

Directions:

Add all the ingredients in the crockpot and cook on LOW heat for 6 to 8 hours.

Stir well and top with shredded cheese.

16. Herb Bread

Servings: 8-10(8-10 loaves)

Preparation Time: 1 hr 45 Minutes

Cooking Time: 2 hrs

Ingredients

3.5 cups or 1/2 pound - bread flour

3.5 cups or 1/2 pound - whole wheat floor

2 packs - dry yeast

2 1/2 cups - warm water

1/2 cup - fresh chopped herbs (basil, rosemary and oregano)

6 tbsps. - extra virgin olive oil

2 tsp - brown sugar

2 tsp - salt

Directions:

Add sugar and to yeast and wait for 10 minutes for it to get frothy.

In a large bowl, mix flours, salt and half the herbs with olive oil. Add little by little and constantly stir until a dough is formed.

Knead it into a smooth ball, cover it and let it rest for an hour.

Once the dough has doubled, roll out the dough and knead it again. Let it sit for 1/2 hour more.

Line crockpot with parchment. Place the dough and brush it with olive oil. Add the remaining herbs and salt on top.

Cook on HIGH for around 2 hours. You can add a paper towel between pot and the lid to catch extra condensation.

Tip: if you want a crispier and browner bread, put it under the broiler for 2-3 minutes.

17. Apple Cinnamon Oatmeal

Servings: 4(4 cups)

Preparation Time: 10 Minutes

Cooking Time: 7-8 hrs

Ingredients

1 Non-stick cooking spray

2 - Large and tart apples (chopped)

1 1/2 cups - skim milk

1 1/2 cups - water

1 cup - whole grain oats

3 tbsps. - Dark brown sugar

2 tbsps. - butter

1 tbsps. - cinnamon

2 tbsps. - flaxseed (ground)

1/4 tsp - kosher salt (as per taste)

Extra toppings

1/4 cup - dried fruit (cranberries and raisins)

1/4 cup - nuts chopped

Directions:

Spray non-stick cooking spray in a crockpot. Mix all ingredients together, except for the kosher salt. Stir mixture well.

Cover and cook on Low setting for 7 or 8 hours (preferably cooked overnight). Add salt to cooked oatmeal and serve.

Serve with extra toppings for added flavour.

Nutrition:

Calories: 321; Fat: 13 g; Carbs: 46 g; Fibre: 6 g; Protein: 7 g

18. Hot Chocolate Steel-Cut Oatmeal

Servings: 4(4 cups)

Preparation Time: 10 Minutes

Cooking Time: 8-9 hrs.

 Ingredients

1 cup - steel-cut oats

4 cup - water

1/2 cup - coconut milk

1 tbsp. - cocoa powder

1 tsp - vanilla

1/4 tsp - salt

1 tbsp. - pure maple syrup or coconut palm sugar

8 drops - liquid stevia (or one tbsp. extra sugar)

Directions:

Combine ingredients in slow cooker and cook at Low setting for 8-9 hours.

Stir the cooked oatmeal before removing to serving bowls.

Nutrition:

Calories: 126; Total Fat: 8 g; Sat Fat: 6.4 g; Sodium:160 mg; Carbs: 12.4 g; Dietary Fiber: 2.1 g, Sugars: 4.4 g; Protein: 2.7 g

19. Oat and whole wheat bread

Servings: 12(12 loaves)

Preparation Time: 15 Minutes

Cooking Time: 3 hrs.

 Ingredients

3/4 packet - yeast

1/4 cup - warm water

1 cup - warm skim milk (1 cup buttermilk)

1/2 cup - rolled oats

1 tsp - salt

2 tbsps. -olive oil

2 tbsps. - honey

1/4 cup - wheat germ

2 3/4 cups - whole wheat flour

Directions:

Grease a glass bowl, 1 lb. coffee can or deep metal pan. Pre-heat crockpot to HIGH.

Dissolve the yeast in water. Add milk, honey, oats, salt, oil, and wheat germ. Add to the frothing yeast mixture.

Add whole wheat flour and knead the dough until it is smooth and elastic. Place dough into greased dish and cover with foil or paper towel.

Add 1/2 cup water to pot and place crumpled foil. Now place the dish in the crockpot. Cover and bake bread on High heat for 3 hours.

Nutrition:

Calories: 163.1; Total Fat: 3.9 g; Sat Fat: 0.7 g; Sodium: 213.7 mg; Carbs: 27.8g; Dietary Fiber: 3.9 g, Sugars: 3 g

20. Pecan Buns

Servings: 12(buns)

Preparation Time: 1 hr. 30 Minutes

Cooking Time: 1 hr15 min. - 1 hr. 30 min. on LOW

Ingredients

Cooking spray

For Dough:

6 tbsps. (90ml) – non-fat milk

4 tbsps. (60ml) - maple syrup

½ tbsp. - unsalted butter (melted)

1 tsp - vanilla extract

¼ tsp - salt

2 ¼ tsp - yeast

180-240g - whole wheat flour

For caramel sauce:

2 tbsps. - unsalted butter

2 tbsps. (30ml) – non-fat milk

4 tbsps. (60ml) - maple syrup

¼ cup - chopped pecans

 For filling:

3 tbsps. (45ml) - maple syrup

1 ½ tsp - ground cinnamon

½ tbsp. - unsalted butter (melted)

Directions:

Coat the pot with cooking spray.

Add butter to pan and melt it on low flame. Remove and add milk, maple syrup and vanilla to the warm, melted butter. Add yeast and let the paste sit for 10 to15 minutes or until it turns frothy.

Add flour, little by little, to the frothy liquid and knead into dough. Let it rest for a while..

Combine butter, milk and maple syrup in a pan. Heat it over medium-low heat and keep stirring until butter melts. When the mixture darkens, remove and add it to the crockpot. Sprinkle pecan nuts on top but leave an inch border around the crockpot's inner rim.

Whisk maple syrup and ground cinnamon in a bowl.

Roll out dough into 10x14 inch length rectangle. Brush the rolled out dough with melted butter and maple-cinnamon filling. Leave ½ inch border on the longer sides. Roll up the dough into a log from one long edge to the other. Slice it into 12 rolls using a dental floss and place each roll over the caramel.

Let the rolls rise for 45 minutes before you cook them on LOW heat for 1 hour 15 to 1 hour 30. Remove cover and let pecan rolls cool for around 10 minutes.

Tip: Don't cool the rolls in the pot for more than 10 minutes as the caramel will harden and the rolls will break when you try to remove them.

Nutrition:

Calories:164; Total Fat: 4.9 g; Sat Fat: 2 g; Unsaturated Fat: 2.4 g; Sodium: 59.4 mg; Carbs: 26.2 g; Dietary Fiber: 2.5 g, Sugars: 11.6 g, Cholesterol: 8.0 mg, Protein: 2.9 g

21. No-Knead Bread

Servings: 1 pound bread (6 -7 loaves)

Preparation Time: 1 hr. 15 Minutes

Cooking Time: 45 min. - 1 hr.

 Ingredients

1/4 tbsp. - granulated yeast

1/4 tbsp. -Kosher salt

1/2 pound (2 cups) - sifted all-purpose flour

200 ml - lukewarm water

Directions:

Pour water in a big bowl and add salt and yeast.

Add the flour and whisk the mixture well. Once it is well mixed, cover the dough, but leave a tiny opening for gases to escape.

Let the dough sit for an hour or until it rises.

Form a ball of the dough and cook in crockpot for 45 to an hour on HIGH. Check for browning after 45 minutes. Press the top of bread. If it is firm to touch, bread has baked well.

Let bread loaf cool on rack before serving.

Tip: for a browner crust, put the bread under broiler for 5 minutes.

22. Apple Butter Sauce

Servings: 4(4 cups)

Preparation Time: 25 Minutes

Cooking Time: 11-13 hrs.

 Ingredients

5 1/2 lbs. - apples (peeled and finely chopped) (use 3-4 varieties)

4 cups - sugar (reduce the sugar by half, if desired)

2 -3 tsp - ground cinnamon

1/4 tsp - ground cloves

1/4 tsp - salt

Directions:

Add apples in large bowl. Mix sugar, salt and spices. Mix well and pour on apples.

Combine well and place apple mixture in crockpot. Cover with lid and cook for 1 hour on HIGH.

Reduce setting to LOW and cook for 9-11 hours. Stir every couple of hours

When sauce thickens and turns dark brown, uncover and cook for another hour

Whisk to make it smoother.

Cool and freeze sauce in airtight containers. Use when required.

Nutrition:

Calories: 154.2; Total Fat: 0.2 g; Sodium: 19.6 mg; Carbohydrate: 40.3 g; Dietary Fiber: 2.7 g; Sugar: 36.4 g; Protein: 0.3 g

23. Mango Madness

PREPARATION TIME: 5 MINUTES

COOKING TIME: 0 MINUTES

SERVES: 4 CUPS

Ingredients

1 banana

1 cup chopped mango (frozen or fresh)

1 cup chopped peach (frozen or fresh)

1 cup strawberries

1 carrot, peeled and chopped (optional)

1 cup water

Directions

Preparing the Ingredients.

Purée everything in a blender until smooth, adding more water if needed.

If you can't find frozen peaches and fresh ones aren't in season, just use extra mango or strawberries, or try cantaloupe.

Per Serving: Calories: 376; Protein: 5g; Total fat: 2g; Carbohydrates: 95g; Fiber: 14g

24. Savory Pancakes

PREPARATION TIME: 10 MINUTES

COOKING TIME: 15 MINUTES

SERVES: 4

Ingredients

1 cup whole-wheat flour

1 teaspoon garlic salt

1 teaspoon onion powder

½ teaspoon baking soda

¼ teaspoon salt

1 cup lightly pressed, crumbled soft or firm tofu

⅓ cup unsweetened plant-based milk

¼ cup lemon juice (about 2 small lemons)

2 tablespoons extra-virgin olive oil

½ cup finely chopped mushrooms

½ cup finely chopped onion

2 cups tightly packed greens (arugula, spinach, or baby kale work great)

Nonstick cooking spray

Directions

Preparing the Ingredients.

In a large bowl, combine the flour, garlic salt, onion powder, baking soda, and salt. Mix well. In a blender, combine the tofu, plant-based milk, lemon juice, and olive oil. Purée on high speed for 30 seconds.

Pour the contents of the blender into the bowl of dry ingredients and whisk until combined well. Fold in the mushrooms, onion, and greens.

Spray a large skillet or griddle pan with nonstick cooking spray and set over medium-high heat. Reduce the heat to medium and add ½ cup of batter per pancake. Cook on both sides for about 3 minutes, or until set. After flipping, press down on the cooked side of the pancake with a spatula to flatten out the pancake. Repeat until the batter is gone.

Divide the cooked pancakes among 4 single-serving containers. Let cool before sealing the lids.

Place the airtight storage containers in the refrigerator for up to 4 days. To reheat, microwave for 1½ to 2 minutes. To freeze, place the pancakes on a parchment paper–lined baking sheet in a single layer. If there's more than one layer, place another piece of parchment paper over the pancakes and place the second layer on top. Place the baking sheet in the freezer for 2 to 4 hours. Transfer the frozen pancakes to a freezer-safe bag (cut the parchment paper and place a small piece between each pancake). To thaw, refrigerate overnight. Preheat an oven or toaster oven to 350ºF. Place the pancakes on a parchment paper–lined baking sheet and bake for 10 to 15 minutes, or stack the pancakes on a plate and microwave for 2 to 3 minutes.

Per Serving: Calories: 246; Protein: 10g; Total fat: 11g; Carbohydrates: 30g; Fiber: 3g

25. Tropi-Kale Breeze

PREPARATION TIME: 5 MINUTES

COOKING TIME: 0MINUTES

SERVES: 4

Ingredients

1 cup chopped pineapple (frozen or fresh)

1 cup chopped mango (frozen or fresh)

½ to 1 cup chopped kale

½ avocado

½ cup coconut milk

1 cup water, or coconut water

1 teaspoon matcha green tea powder (optional)

Directions

Preparing the Ingredients.

Purée everything in a blender until smooth, adding more water (or coconut milk) if needed.

Per Serving: Calories: 566; Protein: 8g; Total fat: 36g; Saturated fat: 1g; Carbohydrates: 66g; Fiber: 12g

26. Tofu-Spinach Scramble

PREPARATION TIME: 20 MINUTES

COOKING TIME: 15 MINUTES

SERVES: 5

Ingredients

1 (14-ounce) package water-packed extra-firm tofu

1 teaspoon extra-virgin olive oil or ¼ cup vegetable broth

1 small yellow onion, diced

3 teaspoons minced garlic (about 3 cloves)

3 large celery stalks, chopped

2 large carrots, peeled (optional) and chopped

1 teaspoon chili powder

½ teaspoon ground cumin

½ teaspoon ground turmeric

½ teaspoon salt (optional)

¼ teaspoon freshly ground black pepper

5 cups loosely packed spinach

Directions

Preparing the Ingredients.

Press and drain the tofu by placing it, wrapped in a paper towel, on a plate in the sink. Place a cutting board over the tofu, then set a heavy pot, can, or cookbook on the cutting board. Remove after 10 minutes. (Alternatively, use a tofu press.)

In a medium bowl, crumble the tofu with your hands or a potato masher. Set aside.

In a large skillet over medium-high heat, heat the olive oil. Add the onion, garlic, celery, and carrots, and sauté for 5 minutes, until the onion is softened.

Add the crumbled tofu, chili powder, cumin, turmeric, salt (if using), and pepper, and continue cooking for 7 to 8 more minutes, stirring frequently, until the tofu begins to brown.

Add the spinach and mix well. Cover and reduce the heat to medium. Steam the spinach for 3 minutes.

Divide evenly among 5 single-serving containers. Let cool before sealing the lids.

Place the containers in the refrigerator for up to 5 days.

Per Serving: Calories: 170; Protein: 7g; Total fat: 9g; Carbohydrates: 9g; Fiber: 3g

27. Chai Chia Smoothie

PREPARATION TIME: 5 MINUTES

COOKING TIME: 0MINUTES

SERVES: 3

Ingredients

1 banana

½ cup coconut milk

1 cup water

1 cup alfalfa sprouts (optional)

1 to 2 soft Medjool dates, pitted

1 tablespoon chia seeds, or ground flax or hemp hearts

¼ teaspoon ground cinnamon

Pinch ground cardamom

1 tablespoon grated fresh ginger, or ¼ teaspoon ground ginger

Directions

Preparing the Ingredients.

Purée everything in a blender until smooth, adding more water (or coconut milk) if needed.

Although dates are super sweet, they don't cause a large blood sugar spike. They're great to boost sweetness while also boosting your intake of fiber and potassium.

Per Serving (3 cups)

Per Serving: Calories: 477; Protein: 7g; Total fat: 29g; Carbohydrates: 57g; Fiber: 14g

28. Banana Bread Rice Pudding

PREPARATION TIME: 5 MINUTES

COOKING TIME: 50 MINUTES

SERVES: 4

Ingredients

1 cup rice

1½ cups water

1½ cups nondairy milk

3 tablespoons sugar (omit if using a sweetened nondairy milk)

2 teaspoons pumpkin pie spice or ground cinnamon

2 bananas

3 tablespoons chopped walnuts or sunflower seeds (optional)

Directions

Preparing the Ingredients.

In a medium pot, combine the rice, water, milk, sugar, and pumpkin pie spice. Bring to a boil over high heat, turn the heat to low, and cover the pot. Simmer, stirring occasionally, until the rice is soft and the liquid is absorbed. White rice takes about 20 minutes; brown rice takes about 50 minutes.

Smash the bananas and stir them into the cooked rice. Serve topped with walnuts (if using). Leftovers will keep refrigerated in an airtight container for up to 5 days.

Per Serving: Calories: 479; Protein: 9g; Total fat: 13g; Saturated fat: 1g; Carbohydrates: 86g; Fiber: 7g

29. Broiled Grapefruit with Cinnamon Pitas

PREPARATION TIME: 10 MINUTES

COOKING TIME: 15 MINUTES

SERVES: 5

Ingredients

2 whole-wheat pitas, cut into wedges

2 tablespoons coconut oil, melted

1 tablespoon ground cinnamon

2 tablespoons brown sugar

1 grapefruit, halved

2 tablespoons pure maple syrup or agave

Directions

Preparing the Ingredients.

Preheat the oven to 375°F.

Line a baking sheet with parchment paper.

Spread pita wedges in a single layer on a baking sheet and brush with melted coconut oil.

In a small bowl, combine the cinnamon and brown sugar and sprinkle over the pita wedges.

Bake in preheated oven until the wedges are crisp, about 8 minutes. Transfer the pita wedges to a plate and set aside.

Turn the oven to broil. Place the grapefruit halves on the baking sheet. Drizzle the maple syrup over the top of the grapefruit, if using. Broil until the syrup bubbles and begins to crystallize, 3 to 5 minutes. Serve immediately.

30. Blueberry Oatmeal Breakfast Bars

PREPARATION TIME: 10 MINUTES

COOKING TIME: 40 MINUTES

SERVES: 12

Ingredients

2 cups uncooked rolled oats

2 cups all-purpose flour

1½ cups dark-brown sugar

1½ teaspoons baking soda

½ teaspoon sea salt

½ teaspoon ground cinnamon

1 cup vegan butter, melted

4 cups blueberries, fresh or frozen

¼ cup organic cane sugar

2 tablespoons cornstarch

Directions

Preparing the Ingredients.

Preheat the oven to 375°F. Lightly grease a 9-by-13-inch baking dish.

In a large bowl, combine the oats, flour, sugar, baking soda, salt, and cinnamon. Add the butter and mix until well incorporated and crumbly.

In a separate large bowl, combine the blueberries, cane sugar, and cornstarch, mixing until the blueberries are evenly coated.

Press 3 cups of the oatmeal mixture into the prepared baking pan. Spread the blueberry mixture on top and crumble the remaining oatmeal mixture over the blueberries.

Bake for 40 minutes.

Remove from the oven and let cool completely before cutting into bars.

31. Chocolate PB Smoothie

PREPARATION TIME: 5 MINUTES

COOKING TIME: 0 MINUTES

SERVES: 4

Ingredients

1 banana

¼ cup rolled oats, or 1 scoop plant protein powder

1 tablespoon flaxseed, or chia seeds

1 tablespoon unsweetened cocoa powder

1 tablespoon peanut butter, or almond or sunflower seed butter

1 tablespoon maple syrup (optional)

1 cup alfalfa sprouts, or spinach, chopped (optional)

½ cup non-dairy milk (optional)

1 cup water

OPTIONAL

1 teaspoon maca powder

1 teaspoon cocoa nibs

Directions

Preparing the Ingredients.

Purée everything in a blender until smooth, adding more water (or non-dairy milk) if needed. Add bonus boosters, as desired. Purée until blended.

Per Serving: Calories: 474; Protein: 13g; Total fat: 16g; Carbohydrates: 79g; Fiber: 18g

32. Orange French Toast

PREPARATION TIME: 15 MINUTES

COOKING TIME: 10 MINUTES

SERVES: 4

Ingredients

3 very ripe bananas

1 cup unsweetened nondairy milk

zest and juice of 1 orange

1 teaspoon ground cinnamon

¼ teaspoon grated nutmeg

4 slices french bread

1 tablespoon coconut oil

Directions

Preparing the Ingredients.

In a blender, combine the bananas, almond milk, orange juice and zest, cinnamon, and nutmeg and blend until smooth. Pour the mixture into a 9-by-13-inch baking dish. Soak the bread in the mixture for 5 minutes on each side.

While the bread soaks, heat a griddle or sauté pan over medium-high heat. Melt the coconut oil in the pan and swirl to coat. Cook the bread slices until golden brown on both sides, about 5 minutes each. Serve immediately.

33. Oatmeal Raisin Breakfast Cookie

PREPARATION TIME: 5 MINUTES

COOKING TIME: 15 MINUTES

SERVES: 2 COOKIES

Ingredients

½ cup rolled oats

1 tablespoon whole-grain flour

½ teaspoon baking powder

1 to 2 tablespoons brown sugar

½ teaspoon pumpkin pie spice or ground cinnamon (optional)

¼ cup unsweetened applesauce, plus more as needed

2 tablespoons raisins, dried cranberries, or vegan chocolate chips

Directions

Preparing the Ingredients.

In a medium bowl, stir together the oats, flour, baking powder, sugar, and pumpkin pie spice (if using). Stir in the applesauce until thoroughly combined. Add another 1 to 2 tablespoons of applesauce if the mixture looks too dry (this will depend on the type of oats used).

Shape the mixture into 2 cookies. Put them on a microwave-safe plate and heat on high power for 90 seconds. Alternatively, bake on a small tray in a 350°F oven or toaster oven for 15 minutes. Let cool slightly before eating.

Per Serving (2 cookies): Calories: 175; Protein: 74g; Total fat: 2g; Saturated fat:0g; Carbohydrates: 39g; Fiber: 4g

34. Berry Beetsicle Smoothie

PREPARATION TIME: 3 MINUTES

COOKING TIME: 0MINUTES

SERVES: 1

Ingredients

½ cup peeled and diced beets

½ cup frozen raspberries

1 frozen banana

1 tablespoon maple syrup

1 cup unsweetened soy or almond milk

Directions

Preparing the Ingredients.

Combine all the ingredients in a blender and blend until smooth.

35. Blueberry Oat Muffins

PREPARATION TIME: 10 MINUTES

COOKING TIME: 20 MINUTES

SERVES: 12 MUFINS

Ingredients

2 tablespoons coconut oil or vegan margarine, melted, plus more for preparing the muffin tin

1 cup quick-cooking oats or instant oats

1 cup boiling water

½ cup nondairy milk

¼ cup ground flaxseed

1 teaspoon vanilla extract

1 teaspoon apple cider vinegar

1½ cups whole-grain flour

½ cup brown sugar

2 teaspoons baking soda

Pinch salt

1 cup blueberries

Directions

Preparing the Ingredients.

Preheat the oven to 400°F.

Coat a muffin tin with coconut oil, line with paper muffin cups, or use a nonstick tin.

In a large bowl, combine the oats and boiling water. Stir so the oats soften. Add the coconut oil, milk, flaxseed, vanilla, and vinegar and stir to combine. Add the flour, sugar, baking soda, and salt. Stir until just combined. Gently fold in the blueberries. Scoop the muffin mixture into the prepared tin, about ⅓ cup for each muffin.

Bake for 20 to 25 minutes, until slightly browned on top and springy to the touch. Let cool for about 10 minutes. Run a dinner knife around the inside of each cup to loosen, then tilt the muffins on their sides in the muffin wells so air gets underneath. These keep in an airtight container in the refrigerator for up to 1 week or in the freezer indefinitely.

Per Serving (1muffin): Calories: 174; Protein: 5g; Total fat: 3g; Saturated fat:2g; Carbohydrates: 33g; Fiber: 4g

36. Quinoa Applesauce Muffins

PREPARATION TIME: 10 MINUTES

COOKING TIME: 15 MINUTES

SERVES: 5

Ingredients

2 tablespoons coconut oil or margarine, melted, plus more for coating the muffin tin

¼ cup ground flaxseed

½ cup water

2 cups unsweetened applesauce

½ cup brown sugar

1 teaspoon apple cider vinegar

2½ cups whole-grain flour

1½ cups cooked quinoa

2 teaspoons baking soda

Pinch salt

½ cup dried cranberries or raisins

Directions

Preparing the Ingredients.

Preheat the oven to 400°F.

Coat a muffin tin with coconut oil, line with paper muffin cups, or use a nonstick tin. In a large bowl, stir together the flaxseed and water. Add the applesauce, sugar, coconut oil, and vinegar. Stir to combine. Add the flour, quinoa, baking soda, and salt, stirring until just combined. Gently fold in the cranberries without stirring too much. Scoop the muffin mixture into the prepared tin, about ⅓ cup for each muffin.

Bake for 15 to 20 minutes, until slightly browned on top and springy to the touch. Let cool for about 10 minutes. Run a dinner knife around the inside of each cup to loosen, then tilt the muffins on their sides in the muffin wells so air gets underneath. These keep in an airtight container in the refrigerator for up to 1 week or in the freezer indefinitely.

Per Serving(1muffin): Calories: 387; Protein: 7g; Total fat: 5g; Saturated fat: 2g; Carbohydrates: 57g; Fiber: 8g

37. Pumpkin Pancakes

PREPARATION TIME: 15 MINUTES

COOKING TIME: 15 MINUTES

SERVES: 4

Ingredients

2 cups unsweetened almond milk

1 teaspoon apple cider vinegar

2½ cups whole-wheat flour

2 tablespoons baking powder

½ teaspoon baking soda

1 teaspoon sea salt

1 teaspoon pumpkin pie spice or ½ teaspoon ground -cinnamon plus ¼ teaspoon grated -nutmeg plus ¼ teaspoon ground allspice

½ cup canned pumpkin purée

1 cup water

1 tablespoon coconut oil

Directions

Preparing the Ingredients.

In a small bowl, combine the almond milk and apple cider vinegar. Set aside.

In a bowl, whisk together the flour, baking powder, baking soda, salt, and pumpkin pie spice. In bowl, combine the almond milk mixture, pumpkin purée, and water, whisking to mix well. Mix the wet ingredients to the dry ingredients and fold together until the dry -ingredients are just moistened.

In a nonstick pan or griddle over medium-high heat, melt the coconut oil and swirl to coat. Pour the batter into the pan ¼ cup at a time and cook until the pancakes are browned, about 5 minutes per side. Serve immediately.

38. Green Breakfast Smoothie

PREPARATION TIME: 10 MINUTES

COOKING TIME: 0 MINUTES

SERVES: 2

Ingredients

½ banana, sliced

2 Cups Spinach or other greens, such as kale

1 Cup sliced berries of your choosing, fresh or frozen

1 orange, peeled and cut into segments

1 cup unsweetened nondairy milk

1 cup ice

Directions

Preparing the Ingredients. In a blender, combine all the ingredients.

Starting with the blender on low speed, begin blending the smoothie, gradually increasing blender speed until smooth. Serve immediately.

39. Blueberry Lemonade Smoothie

PREPARATION TIME: 5 MINUTES

COOKING TIME: 0 MINUTES

SERVES: 1

Ingredients

1 cup roughly chopped kale

¾ cup frozen blueberries

1 cup unsweetened soy or almond milk

Juice of 1 lemon

1 tablespoon maple syrup

Directions

Preparing the Ingredients.

Combine all the ingredients in a blender and blend until smooth. Enjoy immediately.

40. Berry Protein Smoothie

PREPARATION TIME: 5 MINUTES

COOKING TIME: 0 MINUTES

SERVES: 1

Ingredients

1 banana

1 cup fresh or frozen berries

¾ cup water or nondairy milk, plus more as needed

1 scoop plant-based protein powder, 3 ounces silken tofu, ¼ cup rolled oats, or ½ cup cooked quinoa

Additions

 1 tablespoon ground flaxseed or chia seeds

 1 handful fresh spinach or lettuce, or 1 chunk cucumber

coconut water to replace some of the liquid

Directions

Preparing the Ingredients

In a blender, combine the banana, berries, water, and your choice of protein.

Add any addition ingredients as desired. Purée until smooth and creamy, about 50 seconds.

Add a bit more water if you like a thinner smoothie.

Per Serving: Calories: 332; Protein: 7g; Total fat: 5g; Saturated fat: 1g; Carbohydrates: 72g; Fiber: 11g

41. Blueberry and Chia Smoothie

PREPARATION TIME: 10 MINUTES

COOKING TIME: 0 MINUTES

SERVES: 2

Ingredients

2 tablespoons chia seeds

2 cups unsweetened nondairy milk

2 cups blueberries, fresh or frozen

2 tablespoons pure maple syrup or agave

2 tablespoons cocoa powder

Directions

Preparing the Ingredients

Soak the chia seeds in the almond milk for 5 minutes.

In a blender, combine the soaked chia seeds, almond milk, blueberries, maple syrup, and cocoa powder and blend until smooth. Serve immediately.

42. Green Kickstart Smoothie

PREPARATION TIME: 5 MINUTES

COOKING TIME: 0 MINUTES

SERVES: 1

Ingredients

½ avocado or 1 banana

½ cup chopped cucumber, peeled if desired

1 handful fresh spinach or chopped lettuce

1 pear or apple, peeled and cored, or 1 cup unsweetened applesauce

2 tablespoons freshly squeezed lime juice

1 cup water or nondairy milk, plus more as needed

Additions

 ½-inch piece peeled fresh ginger

1 tablespoon ground flaxseed or chia seeds

½ cup soy yogurt or 3 ounces silken tofu

 coconut water to replace some of the liquid

 2 tablespoons chopped fresh mint or ½ cup chopped mango

Directions

Preparing the Ingredients

In a blender, combine the avocado, cucumber, spinach, pear, lime juice, and water.

Add any Additions ingredients as desired. Purée until smooth and creamy, about 50 seconds. Add a bit more water if you like a thinner smoothie.

Per Serving: Calories: 263; Protein: 4g; Total fat: 14g; Saturated fat: 2g; Carbohydrates: 36g; Fiber: 10g

43. Warm Maple and Cinnamon Quinoa

PREPARATION TIME: 5 MINUTES

COOKING TIME: 15 MINUTES

SERVES: 4

Ingredients

1 cup unsweetened nondairy milk

1 cup water

1 cup quinoa, rinsed

1 teaspoon cinnamon

¼ cup chopped pecans or other nuts or seeds, such as chia, sunflower seeds, or almonds

2 tablespoons pure maple syrup or agave

Directions

Preparing the Ingredients

In a medium saucepan over medium-high heat, bring the almond milk, water, and quinoa to a boil. Lower the heat to medium-low and cover. Simmer until the liquid is mostly absorbed and the quinoa softens, about 15 minutes.

Turn off the heat and allow to sit, covered, for 5 minutes. Stir in the cinnamon, pecans, and syrup. Serve hot.

44. Warm Quinoa Breakfast Bowl

PREPARATION TIME: 5 MINUTES

COOKING TIME: 0 MINUTES

SERVES: 4

Ingredients

3 cups freshly cooked quinoa

1⅓ cups unsweetened soy or almond milk

2 bananas, sliced

1 cup raspberries

1 cup blueberries

½ cup chopped raw walnuts

¼ cup maple syrup

Directions

Preparing the Ingredients

Divide the ingredients among 4 bowls, starting with a base of ¾ cup quinoa, ⅓ cup milk, ½ banana, ¼ cup raspberries, ¼ cup blueberries, and 2 tablespoons walnuts.

Drizzle 1 tablespoon of maple syrup over the top of each bowl.

45. Banana Bread Rice Pudding

PREPARATION TIME: 5 MINUTES

COOKING TIME: 50 MINUTES

SERVES: 4

Ingredients

1cup brown rice

1½ cups water

1½ cups nondairy milk

3 tablespoons sugar (omit if using a sweetened nondairy milk)

2 teaspoons pumpkin pie spice or ground cinnamon

2 bananas

3 tablespoons chopped walnuts or sunflower seeds (optional)

Directions

Preparing the Ingredients.

In a medium pot, combine the rice, water, milk, sugar, and pumpkin pie spice. Bring to a boil over high heat, turn the heat to low, and cover the pot. Simmer, stirring occasionally, until the rice is soft and the liquid is absorbed. White rice takes about 20 minutes; brown rice takes about 50 minutes.

Smash the bananas and stir them into the cooked rice. Serve topped with walnuts (if using). Leftovers will keep refrigerated in an airtight container for up to 5 days.

Per Serving: Calories: 479; Protein: 9g; Total fat: 13g; Saturated fat: 1g; Carbohydrates: 86g; Fiber: 7g

46. Apple and Cinnamon Oatmeal

PREPARATION TIME: 10 MINUTES • COOK TIME:10 MINUTES

SERVES: 2

Ingredients

1¼ cups apple cider

1 apple, peeled, cored, and chopped

⅔ cup rolled oats

1 teaspoon ground cinnamon

1 tablespoon pure maple syrup or agave (optional)

Directions

Preparing the Ingredients.

In a medium saucepan, bring the apple cider to a boil over medium-high heat. Stir in the apple, oats, and cinnamon.

Bring the cereal to a boil and turn down heat to low. Simmer until the oatmeal thickens, 3 to 4 minutes. Spoon into two bowls and sweeten with maple syrup, if using. Serve hot.

47. Mango Key Lime Pie Smoothie

PREPARATION TIME: 5 MINUTES

COOKING TIME: 0 MINUTES

SERVES: 1

Ingredients

¼ avocado

1 cup baby spinach

½ cup frozen mango chunks

1 cup unsweetened soy or almond milk

Juice of 1 lime (preferably a Key lime).

1 tablespoon maple syrup

Directions

Preparing the Ingredients.

Combine all the ingredients in a blender and blend until smooth. Enjoy immediately.

48. Spiced Orange Breakfast Couscous

PREPARATION TIME: 10 MINUTES

COOKING TIME: 10 MINUTES

SERVES: 4

Ingredients

3 cups orange juice

1½ cups couscous

1 teaspoon ground cinnamon

¼ teaspoon ground cloves

½ cup dried fruit, such as raisins or apricots

½ cup chopped almonds or other nuts or seeds

Directions

Preparing the Ingredients.

In a small saucepan, bring the orange juice to a boil. Add the couscous, cinnamon, and cloves and remove from heat. Cover the pan with a lid and allow to sit until the -couscous softens, about 5 minutes.

Fluff the couscous with a fork and stir in the dried fruit and nuts. Serve -immediately.

49. Breakfast Parfaits

PREPARATION TIME: 15 MINUTES

COOKING TIME: 0 MINUTES

SERVES: 2

Ingredients

one 14-ounce can coconut milk, refrigerated overnight

1 cup granola

½ cup walnuts

1 cup sliced strawberries or other seasonal berries

Directions

1. Pour off the canned coconut-milk liquid and retain the solids.

2. In two parfait glasses, layer the coconut-milk solids, granola, walnuts, and -strawberries. Serve immediately.

50. Sweet Potato and Kale Hash

PREPARATION TIME: 10 MINUTES

COOKING TIME: 15 MINUTES

SERVES: 2

Ingredients

1 sweet potato

2 tablespoons olive oil

½ onion, chopped

1 carrot, peeled and chopped

2 garlic cloves, minced

½ teaspoon dried thyme

1 cup chopped kale

sea salt

freshly ground black pepper

Directions

Preparing the Ingredients.

1. Prick the sweet potato with a fork and microwave on high until soft, about 5 minutes. Remove from the microwave and cut into ¼-inch cubes.

2. In a large nonstick sauté pan, heat the olive oil over medium-high heat. Add the onion and carrot and cook until softened, about 5 minutes. Add the garlic and thyme and cook until the garlic is fragrant, about 30 seconds.

3. Add the sweet potatoes and cook until the potatoes begin to brown, about 7 -minutes. Add the kale and cook just until it wilts, 1 to 2 minutes. Season with salt and pepper. Serve immediately.

Chapter 4. Lunch recipes

51. Coconut Artichoke Soup

Preparation time: 10 minutes

Cooking time: 30 minutes

Servings: 4

Ingredients:

10 ounces canned artichokes hearts, drained and quartered

2 tablespoons avocado oil

3 scallions, chopped

4 cups veggie stock

14 ounces coconut milk

Salt and black pepper to the taste

3 tablespoons red curry paste

1 tablespoon coriander, chopped

Directions:

Heat up a pot with the oil over medium heat, add the scallions and the curry paste and sauté for 5 minutes.

Add the artichokes and the other ingredients, toss, bring to a simmer and cook over medium heat for 25 minutes more.

Divide soup into bowls and serve.

Nutrition: calories 271, fat 5, fiber 6, carbs 22, protein 6

52. Dill Cucumber Soup

Preparation time: 10 minutes

Cooking time: 0 minutes

Servings: 4

Ingredients:

2 cucumbers, peeled and chopped

2 spring onions, chopped

2 cups coconut cream

4 garlic cloves, minced

1 tablespoon dill, chopped

Juice of 1 lime

A pinch of salt and black pepper

2 cups veggie stock

Directions:

In a blender, combine the cucumber with the onions and the other ingredients, pulse well, divide into bowls and serve cold.

Nutrition: calories 201, fat 4, fiber 6, carbs 13, protein 5

53. Mushroom and Tomato Soup

Preparation time: 10 minutes

Cooking time: 30 minutes

Servings: 6

Ingredients:

4 scallions, chopped

1 tablespoon olive oil

1 pound white mushrooms, sliced

1 cup cherry tomatoes, halved

1 celery stalk, chopped

2 garlic cloves, minced

6 cups veggie stock

A pinch of salt and black pepper

1 tablespoon cilantro, chopped

Directions:

Heat up a pot with the oil over medium heat, add the scallions and the garlic and sauté for 5 minutes.

Add the mushrooms and sauté for 5 minutes more.

Add the rest of the ingredients, toss, bring to a simmer and cook over medium heat for 20 minutes.

Divide the soup into bowls and serve.

Nutrition: calories 212, fat 5, fiber 7, carbs 10, protein 5

54. Mushrooms and Chestnuts Soup

Preparation time: 10 minutes

Cooking time: 30 minutes

Servings: 6

Ingredients:

2 celery stalks, chopped

2 spring onions, chopped

8 ounces water chestnuts, chopped

2 teaspoons garlic, minced

2 tablespoons coconut aminos

1 quart veggie stock

5 ounces white mushrooms, sliced

2 tablespoons olive oil

1 tablespoon cilantro, chopped

Directions:

Heat up a pot with the oil over medium heat, add the onions and the garlic and sauté for 5 minutes.

Add the mushrooms and sauté for 5 minutes more.

Add the rest of the ingredients, toss, cook over medium heat for 20 minutes, divide into bowls and serve.

Nutrition: calories 281, fat 4, fiber 6, carbs 13, protein 4

55. Veggie Stew

Preparation time: 10 minutes

Cooking time: 35 minutes

Servings: 4

Ingredients:

4 scallions, chopped

3 garlic cloves, minced

2 tablespoons olive oil

1 teaspoon coriander, ground

½ teaspoon fennel seeds, crushed

1 teaspoon cumin, ground

A pinch of salt and black pepper

¼ teaspoon cardamom powder

2 cups cauliflower florets

2 cups broccoli florets

1 cup cherry tomatoes, halved

2 ounces tomato passata

1 green bell pepper, chopped

1 red bell pepper, chopped

1 tablespoon cilantro, chopped

Directions:

Heat up a pot with the oil over medium heat, add the scallions and the garlic and sauté for 2 minutes.

Add the coriander, fennel, cumin, salt, pepper and the cardamom and sauté for 3 minutes more.

Add the rest of the ingredients, toss, cook over medium heat for 30 minutes, divide into bowls and serve for lunch.

Nutrition: calories 139, fat 7.7, fiber 5.4, carbs 16.2, protein 4.8

56. Spinach Curry

Preparation time: 10 minutes

Cooking time: 25 minutes

Servings: 4

Ingredients:

1 pound baby spinach

2 garlic cloves, minced

2 tablespoons avocado oil

1 teaspoon chili powder

1 teaspoon cumin, ground

½ cup coconut cream

1 teaspoon turmeric powder

1 cup tomatoes, cubed

1 teaspoon ginger, grated

3 scallions, chopped

1 cup veggie stock

2 tablespoons green curry paste

½ teaspoon coriander powder

A pinch of salt and black pepper

2 tablespoons cilantro, chopped

Directions:

Heat up a pot with the oil over medium heat, add the garlic, scallions, chili, cumin and turmeric and sauté for 5 minutes.

Add the spinach and the other ingredients, toss, cook over medium heat for 20 minutes, divide into bowls and serve.

Nutrition: calories 151, fat 10.9, fiber 4.8, carbs 13.3, protein 5

57. Brussels Sprouts Soup

Preparation time: 10 minutes

Cooking time: 35 minutes

Servings: 4

Ingredients:

4 scallions, chopped

2 garlic cloves, minced

1 tablespoon olive oil

1 pound Brussels sprouts, trimmed and halved

3 teaspoons ginger, grated

A pinch of salt and black pepper

5 cups vegetable stock

1 teaspoon sweet paprika

1 teaspoon cumin, ground

2 teaspoons tomato passata

1 teaspoon coconut aminos

1 tablespoon cilantro, chopped

Directions:

Heat up a pot with the oil over medium heat, add the scallions, ginger and the garlic and sauté for 5 minutes.

Add the sprouts and the other ingredients, toss, bring to a simmer, cook over medium heat for 30 minutes, divide into bowls and serve.

Nutrition: calories 111, fat 4.7, fiber 6.1, carbs 16.2, protein 5.5

58. Okra Soup

Preparation time: 10 minutes

Cooking time: 6 hours

Servings: 8

Ingredients:

1 green bell pepper, chopped

1 red bell pepper, chopped

3 scallions, chopped

4 cups veggie stock

16 ounces okra, sliced

A pinch of salt and black pepper

1 cup cherry tomatoes, cubed

1 teaspoon coriander, ground

1 teaspoon cumin, ground

1 tablespoon tomato passata

1 teaspoon marjoram, dried

1 teaspoon thyme, dried

1 tablespoon oregano, chopped

Directions:

In your slow cooker, combine the peppers with the scallions, the okra and the other ingredients, toss, put the lid on and cook on Low for 6 hours.

Ladle into bowls and serve.

Nutrition: calories 49, fat 1.4, fiber 3.2, carbs 9.9, protein 2.1

59. Okra and Green Beans Soup

Preparation time: 10 minutes

Cooking time: 30 minutes

Servings: 4

Ingredients:

1 pound green beans, trimmed and halved

1 cup okra, sliced

3 scallions, chopped

4 cups veggie stock

2 tablespoons olive oil

1 teaspoon chili powder

1 teaspoon cumin, ground

1 teaspoon coriander, ground

Salt and black pepper to the taste

1 teaspoon thyme, dried

1 cup coconut milk

1 tablespoon cilantro, chopped

Directions:

Heat up a pot with the oil over medium heat, add the scallions, chili powder, cumin, coriander, thyme, salt and pepper and sauté for 5 minutes.

Add the green beans and the other ingredients, toss, .bring to a simmer and cook over medium heat for 25 minutes more.

Divide the soup into bowls and serve.

Nutrition: calories 281, fat 4, fiber 7, carbs 13, protein 5

60. Ginger Cream

Preparation time: 5 minutes

Cooking time: 25 minutes

Servings: 4

Ingredients:

1 cup cucumber, grated

2 tablespoons ginger paste

2 scallions, chopped

1 tablespoon avocado oil

4 cups veggie stock

2 teaspoons curry powder

1 teaspoon turmeric powder

Salt and black pepper to the taste

14 ounces coconut milk

Directions:

Heat up a pot with the oil over medium heat, add the scallions and the ginger paste and sauté for 5 minutes.

Add the cucumber and the other ingredients, bring to a simmer and cook over medium heat for 20 minutes more.

Blend the soup using an immersion blender, divide the soup into bowls and serve.

Nutrition: calories 281, fat 2, fiber 4, carbs 15, protein 7

61. Savoy Cabbage Soup

Preparation time: 10 minutes

Cooking time: 35 minutes

Servings: 4

Ingredients:

2 tablespoons avocado oil

4 scallions, chopped

2 tablespoons balsamic vinegar

2 green chilies, chopped

2 garlic cloves, minced

2 celery stalks, chopped

6 cups vegetable stock

1 Savoy cabbage head, cut into medium strips

1 cup green beans, trimmed and halved

1 tablespoon thyme, chopped

A pinch of salt and black pepper

Directions:

Heat up a pot with the oil over medium heat, add the scallions, chilies and the garlic and sauté for 5 minutes.

Add the celery and the other ingredients, toss, bring to a simmer and cook over medium heat for 30 minutes.

Divide the soup into bowls and serve.

Nutrition: calories 371, fat 8, fiber 12, carbs 28, protein 12

62. Peppers and Hot Cauliflower Soup

Preparation time: 10 minutes

Cooking time: 40 minutes

Servings: 4

Ingredients:

1 pound cauliflower florets

1 red bell pepper, roughly chopped

1 green bell pepper, roughly chopped

1 orange bell pepper, roughly chopped

2 tablespoons avocado oil

2 scallions, chopped

1 cup tomato passata

5 cups veggie stock

½ teaspoon basil, dried

½ teaspoon oregano, dried

1 tablespoon cilantro, chopped

A pinch of salt and black pepper

Directions:

Heat up a pot with the oil over medium heat, add the scallions and the peppers and sauté for 5 minutes.

Add the cauliflower and the other ingredients, toss, bring to a simmer and cook over medium heat for 35 minutes.

Ladle the soup into bowls and serve.

Nutrition: calories 216, fat 6, fiber 6, carbs 18, protein 7

63. Tomato Curry

Preparation time: 5 minutes

Cooking time: 25 minutes

Servings: 4

Ingredients:

1 pound cherry tomatoes, halved

2 garlic cloves, minced

4 scallions, chopped

2 tablespoons olive oil

1 teaspoon curry powder

½ teaspoon turmeric powder

½ teaspoon cumin, ground

1 cup coconut cream

1 tablespoon red curry paste

1 tablespoon cilantro, chopped

Directions:

Heat up a pot with the oil over medium heat, add the scallions and the garlic and sauté for 5 minutes.

Add the tomatoes and the other ingredients, toss, cook over medium heat for 20 minutes more, divide into bowls and serve for lunch.

Nutrition: calories 371, fat 6, fiber 9, carbs 20, protein 16

64. Brussels Sprouts and Cabbage Stew

Preparation time: 10 minutes

Cooking time: 25 minutes

Servings: 4

Ingredients:

1 pounds Brussels sprouts, trimmed

1 small green cabbage head, shredded

2 tablespoons avocado oil

4 scallions, chopped

1 teaspoon sweet paprika

1 teaspoon chili powder

1 cup tomato passata

1 cup vegetable stock

1 tablespoon dill, chopped

Salt and black pepper to the taste

Directions:

Heat up a pot with the oil over medium heat, add the scallions, paprika and chili powder and sauté for 5 minutes.

Add the sprouts, the cabbage and the other ingredients, toss, cook over medium heat for 20 minutes more, divide into bowls and serve for lunch.

Nutrition: calories 121, fat 4, fiber 7, carbs 14, protein 5

65. Turmeric Cabbage And Tomatoes Stew

Preparation time: 10 minutes

Cooking time: 25 minutes

Servings: 4

Ingredients:

2 tablespoons olive oil

4 spring onions, chopped

2 garlic cloves, minced

2 cups cherry tomatoes, halved

1 green cabbage head, shredded

1 cup tomato passata

Salt and black pepper to the taste

1 teaspoon cumin, ground

1 teaspoon coriander, ground

1 tablespoon basil, chopped

2 teaspoons turmeric powder

Directions:

Heat up a pot with the oil over medium heat, add the garlic, spring onions, cumin, coriander and turmeric and sauté for 5 minutes.

Add the cabbage, tomatoes and the other ingredients, toss, cook over medium heat for 20 minutes more, divide into bowls and serve for lunch.

Nutrition: calories 152, fat 5, fiber 8, carbs 9, protein 10

66. Endives and Green Beans Stew

Preparation time: 10 minutes

Cooking time: 30 minutes

Servings: 4

Ingredients:

2 endives, trimmed and shredded

1 pound green beans, trimmed and halved

2 tablespoons avocado oil

2 scallions, chopped

1 teaspoon chili powder

1 teaspoon hot paprika

1 cup tomato passata

Salt and black pepper to the taste

Juice of 1 lime

2 tablespoons parsley, chopped

Directions:

Heat up a pot with the oil over medium heat, add the scallions, chili powder and the paprika and sauté for 5 minutes.

Add the endives and the other ingredients, toss, cook over medium heat for 25 minutes, divide into bowls and serve.

Nutrition: calories 100, fat 4, fiber 7, carbs 9, protein 4

67. Fennel and Rice

Preparation time: 10 minutes

Cooking time: 25 minutes

Servings: 4

Ingredients:

1 cup cauliflower rice

2 fennel bulbs, sliced

2 tablespoons avocado oil

2 scallions, chopped

2 garlic cloves, minced

2 tablespoons tomato passata

1 tablespoon oregano, chopped

1 tablespoon basil, chopped

1 cup veggie stock

3 tablespoons coconut cream

Salt and black pepper to the taste

Directions:

Heat up a pan with the oil over medium heat, add the scallions and the garlic and sauté for 5 minutes.

Add the cauliflower rice, the fennel and the other ingredients, cook over medium heat for 20 minutes, stirring from time to time, divide into bowls and serve for lunch.

Nutrition: calories 264, fat 6, fiber 8, carbs 10, protein 5

68. Tomato Cream

Preparation time: 10 minutes

Cooking time: 20 minutes

Servings: 4

Ingredients:

1 pound cherry tomatoes, halved

4 cups vegetable stock

2 spring onions, chopped

1 teaspoon sweet paprika

½ cup coconut cream

A pinch of salt and black pepper

2 tablespoons avocado oil

1 tablespoon chives, chopped

Directions:

Heat up a pot with the oil over medium heat, add the spring onions and the paprika and sauté for 5 minutes.

Add the tomatoes, stock and the other ingredients except the chives, stir, bring to a simmer and cook for 15 minutes.

Blend the mix using an immersion blender, divide the cream into bowls and serve with the chives sprinkled on top.

Nutrition: calories 111, fat 8, fiber 3.3, carbs 10.2, protein 3.7

69. Cauliflower Stew

Preparation time: 10 minutes

Cooking time: 25 minutes

Servings: 4

Ingredients:

1 pound cauliflower florets

4 scallions, chopped

½ teaspoon cumin, ground

2 tablespoons avocado oil

2 tablespoons tomato passata

2 garlic cloves, minced

A pinch of salt and black pepper

1 cup vegetable stock

1 tablespoon coriander, chopped

Directions:

Heat up a pot with the oil over medium heat, add the scallions and the garlic and sauté for 5 minutes.

Add the cauliflower and the other ingredients, toss, bring to a simmer and cook over medium heat for 20 minutes more.

Divide everything between plates and serve for lunch.

Nutrition: calories 57, fat 1.7, fiber 3.9, carbs 10.7, protein 3.1

70. Seitan Cauliflower Bowl

Preparation Time: 10 minutes

Cooking Time: 22 minutes + 1 hour marinating

Servings: 4

Ingredients:

¼ cup coconut aminos

½ lemon, juiced

3 tsp garlic powder

1 tbsp swerve sugar

1 lb seitan, cut into strips

1 cup olive oil

6 garlic cloves, minced

2 ½ cups cauliflower rice

2 tbsp olive oil

4 large eggs

2 tbsp chopped fresh scallions, for garnishing

Directions:

In a medium bowl, mix the coconut aminos, lemon juice, garlic powder, and swerve sugar.

Add the seitan, coat well in the mix and marinate for 1 hour.

Heat the olive oil in a medium wok and fry the seitan on both sides until brown and cooked through, 10 minutes. Transfer the seitan to a plate and set aside for serving.

Sauté the garlic in the wok until fragrant, 30 seconds. Stir in the cauliflower rice until softened, 5 minutes and season with salt and black pepper. Spoon the food into 4 serving bowls and set aside.

Wipe the wok clean with a paper towel and heat in 1 tablespoon of olive oil.

Crack in two eggs and fry sunshine-style, 1 minute. Place an egg on each cauliflower rice bowl and fry the remaining eggs with the remaining olive oil. Plate also.

Divide the seitan on the food, garnish with some scallions, and serve immediately.

Nutrition:

Calories:823 ,Total Fat: 75.5g, Saturated Fat:14 g, Total Carbs: 8 g, Dietary Fiber: 2g, Sugar:2 g, Protein: 31g, Sodium: 198mg

71. Cheesy Mushroom in Omelet

Preparation Time: 15 minutes

Cooking Time: 20 minutes

Servings: 2

Ingredients:

4 large eggs

2 tbsp almond milk

2 tbsp olive oil

1 medium yellow onion, sliced

½ medium green bell pepper, deseeded and sliced

¼ lb cremini mushrooms, sliced

Salt and black pepper to taste

2 oz provolone cheese, very thinly sliced

Directions:

Beat the eggs with the almond milk in a medium bowl.

Heat half of the olive oil in a medium skillet and pour a quarter of the eggs. Fry until cooked on one side, carefully flip with a spatula, and cook until well-done. Slide onto a plate and make three more eggs. Place on different plates when ready.

Heat the remaining olive oil in the same skillet and sauté the onion and bell pepper until softened, 5 minutes. Transfer to a plate and set aside.

Season the mushrooms with salt and black pepper, add to the skillet, and cook until softened, 5 minutes. Return the onion and pepper to the pan and cook for 1 minute to keep warm. Turn the heat off.

Layer the provolone cheese evenly in the omelet and top with the hot mushroom mixture.

Roll the eggs and place back in the skillet over low heat to melt the cheese.

Transfer to serving plates and serve immediately.

Nutrition:

Calories: 199,Total Fat: 15.7g, Saturated Fat:5.1 g, Total Carbs: 4 g, Dietary Fiber: 1g, Sugar: 2g, Protein: 11g, Sodium: 201mg

72. Cajun Tofu in Mushrooms

Preparation Time: 10 minutes

Cooking Time: 43 minutes

Servings: 4

Ingredients:

2 tbsp olive oil

½ celery stalk, chopped

1 small red onion, finely chopped

1 lb tofu, pressed and crumbled

Salt and black pepper to taste

2 tbsp mayonnaise

1 tsp Cajun seasoning

½ tsp garlic powder

½ cup shredded Gouda cheese

2 large eggs

4 large caps Portobello mushrooms

1 tbsp almond meal

2 tbsp shredded Parmesan cheese

1 tbsp chopped fresh parsley

Directions:

Preheat the oven to 350 F and lightly grease a baking sheet with cooking spray. Set aside.

Heat half of the olive oil in a medium skillet over medium heat and sauté the celery, red onion until softened, 3 minutes. Transfer to a medium mixing bowl.

Add the remaining olive oil to the skillet, season the tofu with salt, black pepper, and cook until brown, 10 minutes. Turn the heat off and transfer to the same bowl.

Pour in the mayonnaise, Cajun seasoning, garlic powder, Gouda cheese, and crack in the eggs. Mix well.

Arrange the mushrooms on the baking sheet and fill with the tofu mix.

In a small bowl, mix the almond meal, Parmesan cheese, and sprinkle on top of the mushroom filling. Cover with foil and bake in the oven until the cheese melts, 30 minutes.

Remove the stuffed mushrooms, take off the foil, and garnish with the parsley.

Serve immediately.

Nutrition:

Calories: 400,Total Fat: 29.1g, Saturated Fat: 8.1g, Total Carbs: 10 g, Dietary Fiber:3 g, Sugar: 2g, Protein:29 g, Sodium: 414mg

73. Braised Seitan with Kelp Noodles

Preparation Time: 10 minutes

Cooking Time: 2 hours 2 minutes

Servings: 4

Ingredients:

1 tbsp olive oil

2 pieces star anise

1 cinnamon stick

1 garlic clove, minced

1-inch ginger, grated

1 ½ lb seitan, cut into strips

3 tbsp tamarind sauce

2 tbsp swerve sugar

¼ cup red wine

¼ cup water

4 cups vegetable broth

2 (23.9oz) kelp noodles, thoroughly rinsed

For topping:

1 cup steamed napa cabbage

Scallions, thinly sliced

Directions:

Heat the olive oil in a medium pot over medium heat and stir-fry the star anise, cinnamon, garlic, and ginger until fragrant, 5 minutes.

Mix in the seitan, season with salt, black pepper, and sear on both sides, 10 minutes.

In a small bowl, combine the tamarind sauce, swerve sugar, red wine, and water. Pour the mixture into the pot, close the lid, and bring to a boil. Reduce the heat and simmer for 30 to 45 minutes or until the seitan is tender.

Strain the pot's content through a colander into a bowl and pour the braising liquid back into the pot. Discard the cinnamon, star anise and set the seitan aside.

Add the vegetable broth to the pot and simmer until hot, 10 minutes.

Put the kelp noodles into the broth and cook until softened and separated, 5 to 7 minutes.

Spoon the noodles with some broth into serving bowls, top with the seitan strips, and then the cabbage and scallions.

Nutrition:

Calories: 311,Total Fat: 18g, Saturated Fat: 6.3g, Total Carbs: 3 g, Dietary Fiber:0 g, Sugar:2 g, Protein:34 g, Sodium:136 mg

74. Stewed Tofu with Walnut Cauliflower Grits

Preparation Time: 15 minutes

Cooking Time: 53 minutes

Servings: 4

Ingredients:

For the stewed tofu:

2 tbsp olive oil

2 lb tofu, cut into 1-inch cubes

Salt and black pepper to taste

1 large yellow onion, chopped

3 garlic cloves, minced

2 large tomatoes, diced

1 tbsp rosemary

1 tbsp smoked paprika

2 tsp chili powder

2 cups vegetable broth

For the walnut cauliflower grits:

2 tbsp butter

½ cup walnuts, chopped

2 cups cauliflower rice

½ cup water

1 cup coconut milk

1 cup shredded provolone cheese

Salt to taste

Directions:

For the stewed tofu:

Heat the olive oil in a large pot over medium heat, season the tofu with salt and black pepper and cook in the oil until brown, 3 minutes.

Stir in the remaining Ingredients and cook over low heat until thickened, 5 to 10 minutes.

Adjust the taste with salt and black pepper, and turn the heat off.

For the walnut cauliflower grits:

Melt the butter in a medium pot and toast in the walnuts for 5 minutes. Transfer to a cutting board, chop and reserve in a plate.

Add the cauliflower rice and water to the pot and cook for 5 minutes or until softened.

Stir in the coconut milk, reduce the temperature, and simmer for 3 minutes.

Mix in the provolone cheese to melt, fold in the walnuts, and adjust the taste with salt.

Spoon the cauliflower grits into serving bowls and top with the stewed tofu.

Nutrition:

Calories: 651,Total Fat: 53.9g, Saturated Fat:23.6 g, Total Carbs: 19 g, Dietary Fiber:5 g, Sugar: 6g, Protein: 32g, Sodium:423 mg

75. Tempeh Zucchini Mug Melt

Preparation Time: 5 minutes

Cooking Time: 2 minutes

Servings: 2

Ingredients:

4 slices cooked tempeh

3 tbsp sour cream

1 small zucchini, chopped

Salt and black pepper to taste

2 tbsp chopped green chilies

3 oz shredded Monterey Jack cheese

Directions:

Divide the tempeh slices in the bottom of two wide mugs and carefully spread with 1 tablespoon of sour cream.

Top with the zucchini, season with salt and black pepper, add the green chilies, and top with the remaining sour cream and then the Monterey Jack cheese.

Place the mugs in the microwave and cook for 1 to 2 minutes or until the cheese melts.

Remove the mugs; allow cooling for 1 minute, and serve.

Nutrition:

Calories:136 ,Total Fat: 9.6g, Saturated Fat: 5.2g, Total Carbs: 5 g, Dietary Fiber: 2g, Sugar: 1g, Protein: 9g, Sodium: 253mg

76. Vegan Sausage with Vegan Bacon

Preparation Time: 5 minutes

Cooking Time: 40 minutes

Servings: 4

Ingredients:

8 large vegan sausages

½ cup grated Swiss cheese

16 slices vegan bacon

1 tsp onion powder

1 tsp garlic powder

Salt and black pepper to taste

Directions:

Preheat the oven to 400 F.

Cut a slit in the middle of each vegan sausage and stuff evenly with the Swiss cheese. Wrap each vegan sausage with 2 vegan bacon slices each and secure with toothpicks. Season with the onion powder, garlic powder, salt, and black pepper.

Place the wrapped vegan sausage on a baking sheet and place in the middle rack of the oven. Cook for 35 to 40 minutes or until the bacon browns and crisps.

Remove the food and serve warm with your preferred side dish.

Nutrition:

Calories:639 ,Total Fat: 55.6g, Saturated Fat:4.6 g, Total Carbs: 9 g, Dietary Fiber: 2g, Sugar: 2g, Protein:28 g, Sodium: 999mg

77. Vegan Sausage Collard Rolls

Preparation Time: 10 minutes

Cooking Time: 1 hour, 3 minutes, 30 seconds

Servings: 4

Ingredients:

1 lb crumbled vegan sausages

1 tbsp butter

Salt and black pepper to taste

2 tsp coconut aminos

1 tsp Dijon mustard

1 tsp whole peppercorns

¼ tsp cloves

¼ tsp allspice

½ tsp red pepper flakes

1 large bay leaf

1 lemon, zested and juiced

¼ cup white wine

¼ cup freshly brewed coffee

2/3 tbsp erythritol

8 large Swiss collard leaves

1 medium red onion, sliced

Directions:

In a large pot, add all the Ingredients up to the collard leaves and mix well.

Close the lid of the pot and cook the Ingredients over low heat for 1 hour or until the vegan sausages cook.

10 minutes to the time being up, boil some water in a medium pot over medium heat and add all the collards with one slice of the onion. Cook for 30 seconds and transfer the leaves immediately to an ice bath to blanch for 5 to 10 minutes.

Remove the collards, pat dry with a paper towel, and lay flat on a flat surface.

Divide the vegan sausages mixture onto the collards, top with the onion slices, and roll the leaves over to cover the filling.

Serve immediately.

Nutrition:

Calories: 356,Total Fat: 21.2g, Saturated Fat: 8.8g, Total Carbs: 10g, Dietary Fiber: 0g, Sugar: 3g, Protein:35 g, Sodium: 557mg

Chapter 5. -Dinner recipes

78. Three Cheese Tofu "Meatza"

Preparation Time: 10 minutes

Cooking Time: 20 minutes

Servings: 4

Ingredients:

1 ½ lb tofu, pressed and crumbled

Salt and black pepper to taste

1 large egg

1 tsp thyme

3 garlic cloves, minced

1 tsp rosemary

1 tsp basil

½ tbsp oregano

¾ cup low-carb tomato sauce

¼ cup shredded Pecorino Romano cheese

1 cup shredded Monterey Jack cheese

1 cup shredded mozzarella cheese

Directions:

Preheat the oven to 350 F and lightly grease a medium pizza pan with cooking spray. Set aside.

In a large bowl, mix the tofu, salt, black pepper, egg, thyme, garlic, rosemary, basil, and oregano.

Transfer the mixture onto the pizza pan and use your hands to flatten the mix onto the pan with 2-inch thickness. Place in the oven and bake for 15 minutes or until the tofu cooks with a light brown crust.

Remove the pizza pan and spread the tomato sauce on top.

Scatter the three cheeses one after the other on top and bake further in the oven until the cheeses melt, 5 minutes.

Remove the "meatza" from the oven, slice, and serve

Nutrition:

Calories:301 ,Total Fat: 25.1g, Saturated Fat: 6.7g, Total Carbs: 5g, Dietary Fiber:1 g, Sugar: 2g, Protein: 15g, Sodium: 669mg

79. Tomatoes and Eggs Plate

Preparation Time: 10 minutes

Cooking Time: 17 minutes

Servings: 4

Ingredients:

5 oz vegan bacon, chopped

1 tbsp olive oil

8 eggs

Salt and black pepper to taste

1 tbsp butter, room temperature

¼ cup red cherry tomatoes

2 tbsp chopped fresh oregano

Directions:

Cook the vegan bacon in a medium skillet over medium heat until brown and crispy, 5 minutes. Divide onto 4 plates and set aside.

Add half of the olive oil into the skillet to heat and crack 4 eggs into the oil. Cook until the egg whites set, but the yolk still runny, 1 minute. Spoon two eggs to the side of the vegan bacon in two plates and fry the remaining eggs using the remaining olive oil. Plate the eggs on two more plates.

Melt the butter in the same skillet, cook in the tomatoes until brown around the edges and a bit on the skin, 8 minutes. Add the egg plates.

Season the food with salt, black pepper, and garnish with the oregano.

Serve warm.

Nutrition:

Calories: 501,Total Fat:43.3 g, Saturated Fat: 21.5g, Total Carbs: 17 g, Dietary Fiber: 5g, Sugar: 7g, Protein18: g, Sodium: 656mg

80. Creamy Cabbage with Tofu and Pine Nuts

Preparation Time: 5 minutes

Cooking Time: 20 minutes

Servings: 4

Ingredients:

For the fried tofu:

2 tbsp butter

25 oz tofu, cut into 6 slabs

For the creamy cabbage:

2 oz butter

25 oz green canon cabbage, shredded

1 ¼ cups heavy cream

½ cup chopped fresh marjoram

Salt and black pepper to taste

½ lemon, zested

2 tbsp toasted pine nuts

Directions:

For the fried tofu:

Melt the butter in a medium skillet over medium heat and fry the tofu on both sides until lightly brown on the outside, 10 minutes. Transfer to a plate and keep warm until ready to serve.

For the creamy cabbage:

Melt the butter in the skillet and sauté the cabbage while occasionally stirring until the cabbage turns golden brown, 4 minutes.

Mix in the heavy cream, allow bubbling, and season with the marjoram, salt, black pepper, and lemon zest.

Divide the tofu onto four plates, spoon the cabbage to the side of the tofu, and sprinkle the pine nuts on the cabbage.

Serve warm.

Nutrition:

Calories:269 ,Total Fat: 21.6g, Saturated Fat: 7.8g, Total Carbs: 6g, Dietary Fiber: 1g, Sugar: 3g, Protein: 13g, Sodium: 298mg

81. Tempeh Mushroom Omelet

Preparation Time: 10 minutes

Cooking Time: 20 minutes

Servings: 2

Ingredients:

2 tbsp olive oil

2 oz tempeh, crumbled

Salt and black pepper to taste

1 small white onion, chopped

¼ cup sliced cremini mushrooms

2 tbsp butter

6 eggs

2 oz shredded cheddar cheese

Directions:

Heat half of the olive oil in a medium frying pan, add the tempeh, season with salt and black pepper, and fry until brown, 10 minutes. Transfer to a plate and set aside.

Heat the remaining olive oil in the pan and sauté the onion and mushrooms until softened, 8 minutes. Spoon to the side of the tempeh and set aside.

Melt the butter in the pan over low heat.

Beat the eggs with some salt, black pepper, and pour into the pan. Swirl to spread the egg around the pan and once the omelet begins to firm, top with the tempeh, mushroom-onion mixture, and cheddar cheese.

Use a spatula to carefully release the egg from around the edges of the pan and flip the egg over the stuffing.

Once beneath the eggs start to golden brown, 2 minutes, slide the eggs onto a serving plate.

Using a knife, divide into half and serve warm.

Nutrition:

Calories:355 ,Total Fat:29.9 g, Saturated Fat:12.5 g, Total Carbs: 4 g, Dietary Fiber:0 g, Sugar: g, Protein: 18g, Sodium: 324mg

82. Seitan Tex-Mex Casserole

Preparation Time: 5 minutes

Cooking Time: 35 minutes

Servings: 4

Ingredients:

2 tbsp butter

1 ½ lb seitan

3 tbsp Tex-Mex seasoning

2 tbsp chopped jalapeño peppers

½ cup crushed tomatoes

Salt and black pepper to taste

½ cup shredded provolone cheese

1 tbsp chopped fresh green onion to garnish

1 cup sour cream for serving

Directions:

Preheat the oven and grease a baking dish with cooking spray. Set aside.

Melt the butter in a medium skillet over medium heat and cook the seitan until brown, 10 minutes.

Stir in the Tex-Mex seasoning, jalapeño peppers, and tomatoes; simmer for 5 minutes and adjust the taste with salt and black pepper.

Transfer and level the mixture in the baking dish. Top with the provolone cheese and bake in the upper rack of the oven for 15 to 20 minutes or until the cheese melts and is golden brown.

Remove the dish and garnish with the green onion.

Serve the casserole with sour cream.

Nutrition:

Calories: 464,Total Fat:37.8 g, Saturated Fat:7.4 g, Total Carbs: 12 g, Dietary Fiber: 2g, Sugar: 3g, Protein:24 g, Sodium: 147mg

83. Tofu Loco Moco

Preparation Time: 12 minutes

Cooking Time: 28 minutes

Servings: 4

Ingredients:

For the loco moco patties:

1 ½ lb tofu, crumbled

1/3 cup almond meal

½ tsp nutmeg powder

1 tsp onion powder

Salt and black pepper to taste

1 large egg

2 tbsp cashew cream

3 tbsp avocado oil

For the mushroom gravy:

1 tbsp salted butter

1 shallot, finely chopped

1 cup sliced oyster mushrooms

1 cup vegetable stock

2 tsp tamarind sauce

Salt and black pepper to taste

½ tsp arrowroot starch

For the fried eggs:

2 tbsp olive oil

4 large eggs

Salt and black pepper to taste

Directions:

For the loco moco patties:

In a large bowl, combine the tofu, almond meal, nutmeg powder, onion powder, salt, and black pepper. In a small bowl, whisk the eggs with the cashew cream and mix into the tofu mixture until the batter is sticky. Form 8 patties from the mixture.

Heat the avocado oil in a medium skillet over medium heat and fry the patties in batches on both sides until compacted and cooked through, 16 minutes. Transfer to a serving plate and set aside.

For the mushroom gravy:

Melt the butter in the same skillet and cook the shallot and mushrooms until softened, 7 minutes.

Meanwhile, in a medium bowl, combine the remaining Ingredients and pour the mixture into the skillet. Cook until slightly thickened, 3 minutes.

Turn the heat off and set aside.

For the fried eggs:

Heat half of the olive oil in a small skillet, crack in an egg, and fry sunshine style, 1 minute. Plate and fry the remaining eggs in the same manner. Season with salt and black pepper.

Serve the tofu with the mushroom gravy and the fried rice.

Nutrition:

Calories: 258,Total Fat: 21g, Saturated Fat: 13.5g, Total Carbs: 16 g, Dietary Fiber: 6g, Sugar: 7g, Protein: 6g, Sodium:37 mg

84. Baked Mushrooms with Creamy Brussels Sprouts

Preparation Time: 8 minutes

Cooking Time: 2 hours 35 minutes

Servings: 4

Ingredients:

For the mushrooms:

1 lb whole white button mushrooms

Salt and black pepper to taste

2 tsp dried thyme

1 bay leaf

5 black peppercorns

½ cups vegetable broth

2 garlic cloves, minced

1 ½ oz fresh ginger, grated

1 tbsp coconut oil

1 tbsp smoked paprika

For the creamy Brussel sprouts:

½ lb Brussel sprouts, halved

1 ½ cups cashew cream

Salt and ground black pepper to taste

Directions:

For the mushroom roast:

Preheat the oven to 200 F.

Pour all the mushroom Ingredients into a baking dish, stir well, and cover with foil. Bake in the oven until softened, 1 to 2 hours.

Remove the dish, take off the foil, and use a slotted spoon to fetch the mushrooms onto serving plates. Set aside.

For the creamy Brussel sprouts:

Pour the broth in the baking dish into a medium pot and add the Brussel sprouts. Add about ½ cup of water if needed and cook for 7 to 10 minutes or until softened.

Stir in the cashew cream, adjust the taste with salt and black pepper, and simmer for 15 minutes.

Serve the creamy Brussel sprouts with the mushrooms.

Nutrition:

Calories: 492,Total Fat: 37.9g, Saturated Fat: 9.1g, Total Carbs: 13g, Dietary Fiber:2 g, Sugar:2 g, Protein: 29g, Sodium: 779mg

85. Pimiento Tofu balls

Preparation Time: 10 minutes

Cooking Time: 15 minutes

Servings: 4

Ingredients:

¼ cup chopped pimientos

1/3 cup mayonnaise

3 tbsp cashew cream

1 tsp paprika powder

1 pinch cayenne pepper

1 tbsp Dijon mustard

4 oz grated Parmesan cheese

1 ½ lbs. tofu, pressed and crumbled

Salt and black pepper to taste

1 large egg

2 tbsp olive oil, for frying

Directions:

In a large bowl, add all the Ingredients except for the olive oil and with gloves on your hands, mix the Ingredients until well combined. Form bite size balls from the mixture.

Heat the olive oil in a medium non-stick skillet and fry the tofu balls in batches on both sides until brown and cooked through, 4 to 5 minutes on each side.

Transfer the tofu balls to a serving plate and serve warm.

Nutrition:

Calories:254 ,Total Fat: 36.8g, Saturated Fat: 8.7g, Total Carbs: 12g, Dietary Fiber: 1g, Sugar: 1g, Protein:26 g, Sodium:773 mg

86. Tempeh with Garlic Asparagus

Preparation Time: 10 minutes

Cooking Time: 18 minutes

Servings: 4

Ingredients:

For the tempeh:

3 tbsp butter

4 tempeh slices

Salt and black pepper to taste

For the garlic buttered asparagus:

2 tbsp. olive oil

2 garlic cloves, minced

1 lb asparagus, trimmed and halved

Salt and black pepper to taste

1 tbsp dried parsley

1 small lemon, juiced

Directions:

For the tempeh:

Melt the butter in a medium skillet over medium heat, season the tempeh with salt, black pepper and fry in the butter on both sides until brown and cooked through, 10 minutes. Transfer to a plate and set aside in a warmer for serving.

For the garlic asparagus:

Heat the olive oil in a medium skillet over medium heat, and sauté the garlic until fragrant, 30 seconds.

Stir in the asparagus, season with salt and black pepper, and cook until slightly softened with a bit of crunch, 5 minutes.

Mix in the parsley, lemon juice, toss to coat well, and plate the asparagus.

Serve the asparagus warm with the tempeh.

Nutrition:

Calories: 181,Total Fat:17.5 g, Saturated Fat:11 g, Total Carbs: 6 g, Dietary Fiber: 3g, Sugar: 2g, Protein: 3g, Sodium: 140mg

87. Mushroom Curry Pie

Preparation Time: 15 minutes

Cooking Time: 55 minutes

Servings 4

Ingredients:

For the piecrust:

1 tbsp flax seed powder + 3 tbsp water

¾ cup coconut flour

4 tbsp chia seeds

4 tbsp almond flour

1 tbsp psyllium husk powder

1 tsp baking powder

1 pinch salt

3 tbsp olive oil

4 tbsp water

For the filling:

1 cup chopped cremini mushrooms

1 cup vegan mayonnaise

3 tbsp + 9 tbsp water

½ red bell pepper, finely chopped

1 tsp turmeric powder

½ tsp paprika powder

½ tsp garlic powder

¼ tsp black pepper

½ cup cashew cream

1¼ cups shredded tofu cheese

Directions:

In two separate bowls, mix the different portions of flax seed powder with the respective quantity of water and set aside to absorb for 5 minutes.

Preheat the oven to 350 F.

Make the crust:

When the flax egg is ready, pour the smaller quantity into a food processor, add the coconut flour, chia seeds, almond flour, psyllium husk powder, baking powder, salt, olive oil, and water. Blend the Ingredients until a ball forms out of the dough.

Line a springform pan with an 8-inch diameter parchment paper and grease the pan with cooking spray.

Spread the dough in the bottom of the pan and bake in the oven for 15 minutes.

Make the filling:

In a bowl, add the remaining flax egg, mushrooms, mayonnaise, water, bell pepper, turmeric, paprika, garlic powder, black pepper, cashew cream, and tofu cheese. Combine the mixture evenly and fill the piecrust. Bake further for 40 minutes or until the pie is golden brown.

Remove, slice, and serve the pie with a chilled strawberry drink.

Nutrition:

Calories:548 ,Total Fat: 55.9g, Saturated Fat:8.5 g, Total Carbs: 6g, Dietary Fiber:2 g, Sugar: 2g, Protein:8 g, Sodium: 405mg

88. Spicy Cheese with Tofu Balls

Preparation Time: 20 minutes

Cooking Time: 20 minutes

Servings: 4

Ingredients:

For the spicy cheese:

1/3 cup vegan mayonnaise

¼ cup pickled jalapenos

1 tsp paprika powder

1 tbsp mustard powder

1 pinch cayenne pepper

4 oz grated tofu cheese

For the tofu balls:

1 tbsp flax seed powder + 3 tbsp water

2 ½ cup crumbled tofu

Salt and black pepper

2 tbsp plant butter, for frying

Directions:

Make the spicy cheese. In a bowl, mix the mayonnaise, jalapenos, paprika, mustard powder, cayenne powder, and cheddar cheese. Set aside.

In another medium bowl, combine the flax seed powder with water and allow absorbing for 5 minutes.

Add the flax egg to the cheese mixture, the crumbled tofu, salt, and black pepper, and combine well. Use your hands to form large meatballs out of the mix.

Then, melt the butter in a large skillet over medium heat and fry the tofu balls until cooked and browned on the outside.

Serve the tofu balls with roasted cauliflower mash and mayonnaise.

Nutrition:

Calories: 259,Total Fat: 55.9g, Saturated Fat:11.4 g, Total Carbs: 5 g, Dietary Fiber: 1g, Sugar: 1g, Protein: 16g, Sodium: 452mg

89. Avocado Coconut Pie

Preparation Time: 30 minutes

Cooking Time: 50 minutes

Servings: 4

Ingredients:

For the piecrust:

1 tbsp flax seed powder + 3 tbsp water

4 tbsp coconut flour

4 tbsp chia seeds

¾ cup almond flour

1 tbsp psyllium husk powder

1 tsp baking powder

1 pinch salt

3 tbsp coconut oil

4 tbsp water

For the filling:

2 ripe avocados

1 cup vegan mayonnaise

3 tbsp flax seed powder + 9 tbsp water

2 tbsp fresh parsley, finely chopped

1 jalapeno, finely chopped

½ tsp onion powder

¼ tsp salt

½ cup cashew cream

1¼ cups shredded tofu cheese

Directions:

In 2 separate bowls, mix the different portions of flax seed powder with the respective quantity of water. Allow absorbing for 5 minutes.

Preheat the oven to 350 F.

In a food processor, add the coconut flour, chia seeds, almond flour, psyllium husk powder, baking powder, salt, coconut oil, water, and the smaller portion of the flax egg. Blend the Ingredients until the resulting dough forms into a ball.

Line a spring form pan with about 12-inch diameter of parchment paper and spread the dough in the pan. Bake for 10 to 15 minutes or until a light golden brown color is achieved.

Meanwhile, cut the avocado into halves lengthwise, remove the pit, and chop the pulp. Put in a bowl and add the mayonnaise, remaining flax egg, parsley, jalapeno, onion powder, salt, cashew cream, and tofu cheese. Combine well.

Remove the piecrust when ready and fill with the creamy mixture. Level the filling with a spatula and continue baking for 35 minutes or until lightly golden brown.

When ready, take out. Cool before slicing and serving with a baby spinach salad.

Nutrition:

Calories:680 ,Total Fat:71.8 g, Saturated Fat:20.9 g, Total Carbs: 10g, Dietary Fiber:7 g, Sugar: 2g, Protein: 3g, Sodium:525 mg

90. Tempeh Coconut Curry Bake

Preparation Time: 7minutes

Cooking Time: 23minutes

Servings: 4

Ingredients:

1 oz. plant butter, for greasing

2 ½ cups chopped tempeh

Salt and black pepper

4 tbsp plant butter

2 tbsp red curry paste

1 ½ cup coconut cream

½ cup fresh parsley, chopped

15 oz. cauliflower, cut into florets

Directions:

Preheat the oven to 400 F and grease a baking dish with 1 ounce of butter.

Arrange the tempeh in the baking dish, sprinkle with salt and black pepper, and top each tempeh with a slice of the remaining butter.

In a bowl, mix the red curry paste with the coconut cream and parsley. Pour the mixture over the tempeh.

Bake in the oven for 20 minutes or until the tempeh is cooked.

While baking, season the cauliflower with salt, place in a microwave-safe bowl, and sprinkle with some water. Steam in the microwave for 3 minutes or until the cauliflower is soft and tender within.

Remove the curry bake and serve with the caulis.

Nutrition:

Calories:417 , Total Fat:38.8g, Saturated Fat:22.4g, Total Carbs: 11g, Dietary Fiber:2g, Sugar: 3g, Protein: 11g, Sodium: 194mg

91. Kale and Mushroom Pierogis

Prep Time:15 minutes

Cooking Time: 30 minutes

Servings: 4

Ingredients:

For the stuffing:

2 tbsp butter

2 garlic cloves, finely chopped

1 small red onion, finely chopped

3 oz. baby bella mushrooms, sliced

2 oz. fresh kale

½ tsp salt

¼ tsp black pepper

½ cup cashew cream

2 oz. grated tofu cheese

For the pierogi:

1 tbsp flax seed powder + 3 tbsp water

½ cup almond flour

4 tbsp coconut flour

½ tsp salt

1 tsp baking powder

1½ cups shredded tofu cheese

5 tbsp butter

Olive oil for brushing

Directions:

Put the butter in a skillet and melt over medium heat, then add and sauté the garlic, red onion, mushrooms, and kale until the mushrooms brown.

Season the mixture with salt and black pepper and reduce the heat to low. Stir in the cashew cream and tofu cheese and simmer for 1 minute. Turn the heat off and set the filling aside to cool.

Make the pierogis: In a small bowl, mix the flax seed powder with water and allow sitting for 5 minutes.

In a bowl, combine the almond flour, coconut flour, salt, and baking powder.

Put a small pan over low heat, add, and melt the tofu cheese and butter while stirring continuously until smooth batter forms. Turn the heat off.

Pour the flax egg into the cream mixture, continue stirring, while adding the flour mixture until a firm dough forms.

Mold the dough into four balls, place on a chopping board, and use a rolling pin to flatten each into ½ inch thin round pieces.

Spread a generous amount of stuffing on one-half of each dough, then fold over the filling, and seal the dough with your fingers.

Brush with olive oil, place on a baking sheet, and bake for 20 minutes or until the pierogis turn a golden brown color.

Serve the pierogis with a lettuce tomato salad.

Nutrition:

Calories:364 , Total Fat:33.4 g, Saturated Fat:17.3 g, Total Carbs:8g, Dietary Fiber:2g, Sugar:3 g, Protein:12 g, Sodium:779 mg

92. Mushroom Lettuce Wraps

Preparation Time: 5minutes

Cooking Time: 16minutes

Servings: 4

Ingredients:

2 tbsp butter

4 oz. baby bella mushrooms, sliced

1½ lbs. tofu, crumbled

½ tsp salt

¼ tsp black pepper

1 iceberg lettuce, leaves extracted

1 cup shredded cheddar cheese

1 large tomato, sliced

Directions:

Put the butter in a skillet and melt over medium heat. Add the mushrooms and sauté until browned and tender, about 6 minutes. Transfer the mushrooms to a plate and set aside.

Add the tofu to the skillet, season with salt and black pepper, and cook until brown, about 10 minutes. Turn the heat off.

Spoon the tofu and mushrooms into the lettuce leaves, sprinkle with the cheddar cheese, and share the tomato slices on top.

Serve the burger immediately.

Nutrition:

Calories:439 , Total Fat:31.9 g, Saturated Fat:12.2 g, Total Carbs: 9 g, Dietary Fiber:4g, Sugar:1 g, Protein:36g, Sodium: 574mg

93. Tofu and Spinach Lasagna with Red Sauce

Preparation Time: 20 minutes

Cooking Time: 45 minutes

Servings: 4

Ingredients:

2 tbsp butter

1 white onion, chopped

1 garlic clove, minced

2 ½ cups crumbled tofu

3 tbsp tomato paste

½ tbsp dried oregano

1 tsp salt

¼ tsp ground black pepper

½ cup water

1 cup baby spinach

Keto pasta

Flax egg: 8 tbsp flax seed powder + 1 ½ cups water

1 ½ cup dairy-free cashew cream

1 tsp salt

5 tbsp psyllium husk powder

Cheese topping

2 cups coconut cream

5 oz. shredded mozzarella cheese

2 oz. grated tofu cheese

½ tsp salt

¼ tsp ground black pepper

½ cup fresh parsley, finely chopped

Directions:

Melt the butter in a medium pot over medium heat. Then, add the white onion and garlic, and sauté until fragrant and soft, about 3 minutes.

Stir in the tofu and cook until brown. Mix in the tomato paste, oregano, salt, and black pepper.

Pour the water into the pot, stir, and simmer the Ingredients until most of the liquid has evaporated.

While cooking the sauce, make the lasagna sheets. Preheat the oven to 300 F and mix the flax seed powder with the water in a medium bowl to make flax egg. Allow sitting to thicken for 5 minutes.

Combine the flax egg with the cashew cream and salt. Add the psyllium husk powder a bit at a time while whisking and allow the mixture to sit for a few more minutes.

Line a baking sheet with parchment paper and spread the mixture in. Cover with another parchment paper and use a rolling pin to flatten the dough into the sheet.

Bake the batter in the oven for 10 to 12 minutes, remove after, take off the parchment papers, and slice the pasta into sheets that fit your baking dish.

In a bowl, combine the coconut cream and two-thirds of the mozzarella cheese. Fetch out 2 tablespoons of the mixture and reserve.

Mix in the tofu cheese, salt, black pepper, and parsley. Set aside.

Grease your baking dish with cooking spray and lay in one-third of the pasta sheet; spread half of the tomato sauce on top, add another one-third set of the pasta sheets, the remaining tomato sauce and the rest of the pasta sheets.

Grease your baking dish with cooking spray, layer a single line of pasta in the dish, spread with some tomato sauce, 1/3 of the spinach, and ¼ of the coconut cream mixture. Season with salt and black pepper as desired.

Repeat layering the Ingredients twice in the same manner making sure to top the final layer with the coconut cream mixture and the reserved cashew cream.

Bake in the oven for 30 minutes at 400 F or until the lasagna has a beautiful brown surface.

Remove the dish; allow cooling for a few minutes, and slice.

Serve the lasagna with a baby green salad.

Nutrition:

Calories:767 , Total Fat:69.8 g, Saturated Fat:34.5 g, Total Carbs:14g, Dietary Fiber:3g, Sugar: 5g, Protein:28 g, Sodium:1205 mg

94. Green Avocado Carbonara

Preparation Time: 15minutes

Cooking Time: 15minutes

Servings: 4

Ingredients:

8 tbsp flax seed powder + 1 ½ cups water

1 ½ cups dairy-free cashew cream

1 tsp salt

5 ½ tbsp psyllium husk powder

Avocado sauce

1 avocado, peeled and pitted

1 ¾ cups coconut cream

Juice of ½ lemon

1 teaspoon onion powder

½ teaspoon garlic powder

¼ cup olive oil

¾ teaspoon sea salt

¼ teaspoon black pepper

Walnut Parmesan or store-bought parmesan

For serving

4 tbsp toasted pecans

½ cup freshly grated tofu cheese

Directions:

Preheat the oven to 300 F.

In a medium bowl, mix the flax seed powder with water and allow sitting to thicken for 5 minutes.

Add the cashew cream, salt, and psyllium husk powder. Whisk until smooth batter forms.

Line a baking sheet with parchment paper, pour in the batter and cover with another parchment paper. Use a rolling pin to flatten the dough into the sheet.

Place in the oven and bake for 10 to 12 minutes. Remove the pasta after, take off the parchment papers and use a sharp knife to slice the pasta into thin strips lengthwise. Cut each piece into halves, pour into a bowl, and set aside.

For the avocado sauce, in a blender, combine the avocado, coconut cream, lemon juice, onion powder, and garlic powder. Puree the Ingredients until smooth.

Pour the olive oil over the pasta and stir to coat properly. Pour the avocado sauce on top and mix. Then, season with salt, black pepper, and the soy cheese. Combine again.

Divide the pasta into serving plates, garnish with extra soy cheese and pecans, and serve immediately.

Nutrition:

Calories:941, Total Fat:94.2g, Saturated Fat:30.4g, Total Carbs:19g, Dietary Fiber:8g, Sugar:5g, Protein:16g, Sodium:1314mg

95. Cashew Buttered Quesadillas with Leafy Greens

Preparation Time: 10minutes

Cooking Time: 20minutes

Servings: 4

Ingredients:

Tortillas

3 tbsp flax seed powder + ½ cup water

½ cup dairy-free cashew cream

1½ tsp psyllium husk powder

1 tbsp coconut flour

½ tsp salt

Filling

1 tbsp cashew butter, for frying

5 oz. grated cheddar cheese

1 oz. leafy greens

Directions:

Preheat the oven to 400 F.

In a bowl, mix the flax seed powder with water and allow sitting to thicken for 5 minutes.

After, whisk the cashew cream into the flax egg until the batter is smooth.

In another bowl, combine the psyllium husk powder, coconut flour, and salt. Add the flour mixture to the flax egg batter and fold in until fully incorporated. Allow sitting for a few minutes.

Then, line a baking sheet with parchment paper and pour in the mixture. Spread into the baking sheet using a spatula and bake in the upper rack of the oven for 5 to 7 minutes or until brown around the edges. Keep a watchful eye on the tortillas to prevent burning.

Remove when ready and slice into 8 pieces. Set aside.

For the filling, spoon a little cashew butter into a skillet and place a tortilla in the pan. Sprinkle with some cheddar cheese, leafy greens, and cover with another tortilla.

Brown each side of the quesadilla for 1 minute or until the cheese melts. Transfer to a plate.

Repeat assembling the quesadillas using the remaining cashew butter.

Serve immediately with avocado salad.

Nutrition:

Calories:224, Total Fat:20.4g, Saturated Fat:12.2g, Total Carbs: 1g, Dietary Fiber:0g, Sugar:1g, Protein:9g, Sodium:556mg

96. Zucchini Boats with Cheese

Preparation Time: 3minutes

Cooking Time: 4minutes

Servings: 2

Ingredients:

1 medium-sized zucchini

4 tbsp butter

2 garlic cloves, minced

1½ oz. baby kale

Salt and black pepper to taste

2 tbsp unsweetened tomato sauce

1 cup cheese

Olive oil for drizzling

Directions:

Preheat the oven to 375 F.

Use a knife to slice the zucchini in halves and scoop out the pulp with a spoon into a plate. Keep the flesh.

Grease a baking sheet with cooking spray and place the zucchini boats on top.

Put the butter in a skillet and melt over medium heat. Add and sauté the garlic until fragrant and slightly browned, about 4 minutes.

Add the kale and the zucchini pulp. Cook until the kale wilts; season with salt and black pepper.

Spoon the tomato sauce into the boats and spread to coat the bottom evenly. Then, spoon the kale mixture into the zucchinis and sprinkle with the cheese.

Bake in the oven for 20 to 25 minutes or until the cheese has a beautiful golden color.

Plate the zucchinis when ready, drizzle with olive oil, and season with salt and black pepper.

Serve immediately.

Nutrition:

Calories:721, Total Fat:76.8g, Saturated Fat:21.2g, Total Carbs: 2g, Dietary Fiber:0g, Sugar:0g, Protein:9g, Sodium:309mg

97. Tempeh Garam Masala Bake

Preparation Time: 5minutes

Cooking Time: 24minutes

Servings: 4

Ingredients:

3 tbsp butter

3 cups tempeh slices

Salt

2 tbsp garam masala

1 green bell pepper, finely diced

1¼ cups coconut cream

1 tbsp fresh cilantro, finely chopped

Directions:

Preheat the oven to 400 F.

Place a skillet over medium heat, add, and melt the butter. Meanwhile, season the tempeh with some salt. Fry the tempeh in the butter until browned on both sides, about 4 minutes.

Stir half of the garam masala into the tempeh until evenly mixed; turn the heat off.

Transfer the tempeh with the spice into a baking dish.

Then, in a small bowl, mix the green bell pepper, coconut cream, cilantro, and remaining garam masala.

Pour the mixture over the tempeh and bake in the oven for 20 minutes or until golden brown on top.

Garnish with cilantro and serve with some cauli rice.

Nutrition:

Calories:286, Total Fat:27g, Saturated Fat:15g, Total Carbs: 5g, Dietary Fiber:0g, Sugar:1g, Protein:9g, Sodium:87mg

98. Caprese Casserole

Preparation Time: 5minutes

Cooking Time: 20minutes

Servings: 4

Ingredients:

1 cup cherry tomatoes, halved

1 cup mozzarella cheese, cut into small pieces

2 tbsp basil pesto

1 cup vegan mayonnaise

2 oz. tofu cheese

Salt and black pepper

1 cup arugula

4 tbsp olive oil

Directions:

Preheat the oven to 350 F.

In a baking dish, mix the cherry tomatoes, mozzarella, basil pesto, mayonnaise, half of the tofu cheese, salt, and black pepper.

Level the Ingredients with a spatula and sprinkle the remaining tofu cheese on top. Bake for 20 minutes or until the top of the casserole is golden brown.

Remove and allow cooling for a few minutes. Slice and dish into plates, top with some arugula and drizzle with olive oil. Serve.

Nutrition:

Calories:588, Total Fat:59g, Saturated Fat:11g, Total Carbs: 2g, Dietary Fiber:1g, Sugar:1g, Protein:13g, Sodium: 646mg

99. Veggie Balls

Preparation time: 40 minutes

Servings: 4 portions:

1 large onion, finely chopped

½ cup sunflower or rapeseed oil for frying

1 red bell pepper, finely chopped

 2 carrots, finely chopped

2-3 cloves garlic, minced

1 cup kale, chopped or minced

12 Oz. cauliflower, minced

2 tbsp. extra virgin olive oil

1 tbsp. vegetable stock powder

½ cup almond or whole-wheat flour

Flour mixed with linen and sesame seeds for dusting

Salt and pepper, to taste

Directions:

• Boil the cauliflower for 5 minutes and then drain. In a food-processor blend it with the extra virgin olive oil until smooth.

• Cook the onion with garlic in a preheated saucepan over medium heat for a minute.

• Add carrots to onion, pepper, cooked peas and kale. Let it cook over a medium heat.

• Add some stock powder, gram flour and season thoroughly with salt and pepper. Mix all the ingredients and remove from heat.

• Sprinkle your hands and chopping board with a little flour mixed with linen and sesame seeds.

• Roll the teaspoon-size mixture into the balls and place them onto the board. You might have about 20 vegetarian "meatballs".

• Pour some oil into the frying pan with seed or sunflower oil, and fry the meatballs, turning them until they are golden-brown all over. Remove from the frying pan to a plate with a kitchen towel/paper to drain the extra virgin olive oil.

Serve the meatballs with the sauce you prefer poured over the top, with any hot dish you prefer.

100. Grilled Vegetable Rolls

Preparation time: 20 minutes

Servings: 4 portions:

For the aubergines:

3 medium aubergines

1 tsp. cumin seeds, toasted

1 pinch of salt

4 ½ tbsp. extra virgin olive oil

For the quinoa and paneer filling:

3½ Oz. feta cheese, grated

3 ½ Oz. paneer, grated

1 small onion, chopped

1 tsp. ginger-garlic paste

¼ tsp. turmeric, ground

1 tsp. garam masala powder

¼ bunch coriander, chopped

1 dash vegetable oil

1 tsp. salt

1 pinch sesame seeds

For the crunchy vegetables:

1 red beetroot, coarsely grated

2 carrots, coarsely grated

1 red pepper, cut small

Directions:

• Combine 3 ½ tablespoons of extra virgin olive oil, the toasted cumin and salt in a bowl, then mix together to make the marinade.

• Cut the top off of the aubergines before cutting lengthways into 4mm thick slices. Brush the aubergine slices with the marinade. Aubergine are thirsty vegetables - they soak up a lot of oil and dry out and crisp up easily, which in this case we don't want, so brush with more oil if necessary.

• Add a tablespoon of extra virgin olive oil to a large frying pan or griddle pan and set over a medium heat. When the oil is hot, add some of the aubergine slices and fry for 2-3 minutes on each side until they soften and have a nice golden colour, then lay them out on some kitchen paper to absorb any excess moisture. Continue to cook in batches until all of the slices are ready.

• To make the paneer and feta cheese filling, add a dash of vegetable oil to a nonstick pan and place over medium heat. When the oil is hot, add the chopped onion and fry until golden.

• Stir in the ginger-garlic paste, ground turmeric andsalt and fry for 2 minutes more.

• Add the feta cheese, cook for 5-7 minutes then sprinkle in the grated paneer. Stir, remove from the heat then sprinkle over the garam masala powder and chopped coriander.

• To assemble, lay out the grilled aubergine slices on a chopping board. Spread a generous layer of the paneer and Feta cheese filling on top of each and sprinkle over the beetroot, carrot and red pepper. Wrap each slice around the filling to create a roll.

Stack the rolls onto a large plate and serve immediately.

101. Baked Eggplant with Cheese

Preparation time: 30 minutes

Servings: 4 portions:

3 tbsp. extra virgin olive oil

2 eggplants, halved lengthways

4 tomatoes

5 Oz. ball mozzarella, drained

1 handful of basil leaves

Salt and pepper, to taste

1 pinch sunflower seeds

Directions:

• Drizzle the oil over the eggplant and bake in the preheated oven (to 200C/fan 180C) for 25 minutes until softened.

• Meanwhile, slice the tomatoes and mozzarella, then arrange on top of the eggplant.

• Return to oven for another 5 mins or until the cheese has melted.

• Scatter over some basil leaves.

Serve with couscous and green salad with the sunflower seeds.

102. Eggplant Pasta

Preparation time: 40 minutes

Servings: 4 portions:

1 pound large eggplant,

1 tbsp. extra virgin olive oil

¼ tsp. garlic, minced

¼ tsp. red pepper flakes

1 small tomato, seeded and chopped

3 tbsp. heavy cream

1 tbsp. basil, chiffonade

2 tbsp. parmesan cheese, grated

1 tbsp. breadcrumbs

¼ cup pomegranate seeds

Kosher salt

Directions:

Peel the eggplant, leaving 1-inch of skin at the top and bottom. Slice the eggplant lengthwise into ¼-inch-thick slices. (I would use a mandolin for this.) Place the eggplant slices on a cooling rack set over the sink and generously sprinkle with kosher salt. Wait 15 minutes, flip, sprinkle again and wait another 15 minutes. Rinse thoroughly under cool water and gently squeeze out excess water. Place on paper towels and pat dry, then cut the slices into ¼-inch-wide strips so that they resemble linguine. Heat a 10-inch sauté pan over medium-high heat and add the oil. When it shimmers, add the garlic and red pepper flakes and toss for 10 seconds. Add the eggplant and toss to coat. Add the tomato and toss for 15 to 20 seconds. Add the cream and toss for another 10 seconds. Finish with the basil and parmesan.

Transfer to a serving dish, top with breadcrumbs. Sprinkle the pomegranate seeds, toss and serve immediately.

103. Stuffed Zucchini

Preparation time: 30 minutes

Servings: 4 portions:

2 zucchini cut in length and cored (boat-shaped)

5 canned, pitted black olives, sliced

3 Oz. of feta cheese for the filling

5 Oz. of finely chopped parmesan or any cheese to liking for seasoning

½ of a medium-size onion, chopped

Zucchini kernel

3 tbsp. of extra virgin olive oil

3 tbsp. of chopped celeriac

7 Oz. cherry tomatoes

Salt, pepper and garlic to liking

1 pinch of dill weed or any herb to liking

Directions:

• Oil and season empty zucchini boats with salt and pepper.

• Stuff zucchini boats in layers with chopped celeriac, feta cheese, chopped onion.

• Add sliced black olives on top.

• Add upper layer with parmesan cheese.

• Pour some extra virgin olive oil and add some salt, pepper and herbs if you like.

• Bake the stuffed zucchini for 10 minutes in a preheated to 350°F/180°C oven.

Serve with fresh Cherry tomatoes.

104. Baked Vegetables with Béchamel Sauce

Preparation time: 30 minutes

Servings: 4 portions:

1 cup salsify, preferably canned

1 cup brussels sprouts

3 carrots, chopped

1 medium potato, cut coarsely

Broccoli or cauliflower, etc., to taste

Béchamel sauce:

2 tbsp. butter

2 tbsp. whole wheat flour

1 cup milk

1 tsp. nutmeg, grated

Salt, pepper, to taste

On top:

½ cup cheddar cheese, grated

Directions:

• Steam all the vegetables and set aside. You might need to cook them separately as the cooking time for every vegetable varies. I zap them in the microwave for a few minutes.

• Melt butter in a saucepan. Add the flour and mix it well. Cook on low heat for about 4-5 minutes, without allowing the flour to turn brown. I take my pan off the burner a few times when doing this in order to avoid browning of the flour.

• Stirring constantly, slowly add the milk in a thin stream and in small batches. (Here's what I do to avoid lumps in my white sauce - transfer the flour from the pan into a mug and add a little milk and mix it thoroughly. Then transfer it back to the pan and add the rest of the milk. The result? Completely lump-free sauce).

• Keep stirring and bring to a boil. Reduce the heat, add all the salt, pepper powder and the mustard paste.

• Finally add the cheese slices and mix well till the cheese melts. Simmer for a few more minutes till the sauce thickens.

• Arrange the vegetables in a baking dish, I use my 9" pie dish. Pour the sauce over it, sprinkle the grated cheese over it and bake in the oven (pre-heat the oven first) at 200 degrees C till the cheese starts to brown.

Serve with some brown whole wheat bread.

105. Low-Carb Mushroom Cauliflower Risotto

Preparation time: 30 minutes

Servings: 4 portions:

6 medium portobello mushrooms

1 cup vegetable broth

2 cups cauliflower, riced

¼ cup heavy cream

½ cup parmesan cheese

1 tbsp. extra virgin olive oil

2 cloves garlic

Salt and pepper to taste

Directions:

• In a food processor, process the cauliflower florets until they become the size of rice.

• In a pan or small pot, cook garlic and mushrooms in a tablespoon of extra virgin olive oil.

• When the garlic is fragrant, add vegetable broth and your riced cauliflower.

• Stir well over the low heat so that the whole dish simmers and cover. Let steam for 10 minutes.

• After it is cooked, let half of the vegetable broth evaporate in an opened pan and cook the cauliflower about 5-10 minutes more. When stirred, add the heavy cream, parmesan cheese and spices to your cauliflower rice.

Stir until parmesan has melted and serve.

106. Baked Spicy Potatoes

Preparation time: 10 minutes

Servings: 4

Ingredients:

2 ½ pounds potatoes (or 3 pounds for less spicy potatoes)

2 tbsp. olive oil

2 garlic cloves, minced (or maybe 1/2 tsp. garlic powder)

2 tsp. parsley, dried

1/2 tsp. cayenne

1/2 tsp. paprika

3/4 tsp. salt

1/2 tsp. pepper

Directions:

Preheat the oven to 450°F or 230°C. Pour the olive oil onto a rimmed cookie sheet. Add the spices and mix with the olive oil. Clean the potatoes and slice them into even wedges. Put the potatoes on the cookie sheet and use your hands to coat the potatoes with the olive oil mix. The baking time will vary depending on how big your wedges are. I usually bake mine for 20 minutes, take them out of the oven to flip them, and bake for another 10 – 15 minutes. If you want them crispier, just bake them for a few minutes longer.

107. Baked Sweet Potatoes

Preparation time: 5 minutes

Servings: 4

Ingredients:

4 medium sweet potatoes, scrubbed

Directions:

Preheat the oven to 425ºF or 220ºC. Scrub sweet potatoes and pierce in several places with a sharp knife. Line a baking sheet with foil and place the potatoes on top. Bake for 45 minutes to an hour, depending on the size of the potatoes, until thoroughly soft and beginning to ooze. Remove from the heat.

Place on a plate or in a dish and allow to cool. Cover with plastic wrap and refrigerate (they will continue to ooze and sweeten). Serve cold (cut and remove the skin) or room temperature, or reheat for 20 to 30 minutes in a 350ºF or 175ºC oven.

108. Fried Vegetables

Preparation time: 15 minutes

Servings: 4

Ingredients:

1 tbsp. olive oil

1 medium onion, sliced thin

1 cup carrots, diagonally sliced

2 cups broccoli florets

2 cups sugar snap peas

1 large red bell pepper, cut into strips

1 tbsp. reduced sodium soy sauce

1 tsp. garlic powder

1 tsp. ginger, ground

2 tsp. sesame seed, toasted

salt and pepper, to taste

Directions:

Heat the oil in wok or large deep skillet on medium-high heat.

Add onion and carrots; stir fry 2 minutes.

Add remaining vegetables; stir fry 5 to 7 minutes or until vegetables are tender-crisp.

Add soy sauce, garlic powder and ginger; stir-fry until well blended.

Sprinkle with sesame seed. Serve over cooked rice, if desired.

109. Curried Couscous with Vegetables

Preparation time: 15 minutes

Servings: 4

Ingredients:

1 large onion, cut in thin wedges

2 cups yellow summer squash and/or zucchini (2 medium), coarsely chopped

2½ oz. can tomatoes with jalapeno peppers, diced

2 cups water

2 5.7 oz. packages curry-flavor couscous mix

1 cup almonds, chopped toasted slivered

1/2 cup raisins (optional)

cilantro sprigs (optional)

salt and pepper, to taste

Directions:

In a 3½ or 4 quart slow cooker, combine onion, summer squash, undrained tomatoes, the water, and the seasoning packets from couscous mixes.

Cover and cook on low-heat setting for 4 to 6 hours or on high-heat setting for 2 to 3 hours.

Stir in couscous.

Turn off cooker.

Cover and let stand for 5 minutes.

Fluff couscous mixture with a fork.

To serve, sprinkle each serving with almonds and raisins.

110. Grilled Vegetables

Preparation time: 10 minutes

Servings: 4

Ingredients:

1 lb. cremini mushrooms, cleaned

2 cups cauliflower, cut into small florets

2 cups cocktail tomatoes

12 cloves garlic, minced

2 tbsp. olive oil

salt and pepper to taste

1 tbsp. fresh parsley, chopped

1 tsp. fresh Italian parsley leaves, chopped

1 tsp. basil leaves, chopped fresh

1/2 tsp. fresh rosemary leaves, finely chopped

Directions:

Preheat oven to 400°F or 200°C. In a bowl add all the mushrooms and veggies. Drizzle with olive oil then add fresh Italian parsley leaves, fresh basil leaves, fresh rosemary leaves, salt, pepper and toss until well combined. Dump the veggies onto a baking sheet and place in the preheated oven. Roast for 20 to 30 minutes or until mushrooms are golden brown and cauliflower is fork tender. Garnish with fresh parsley before serving.

111. Stewed Beans in Tomato Sauce

Preparation time: 10 minutes

Servings: 4

Ingredients:

1 lb. dried white beans, such as Great Northern or cannellini, picked over, rinsed, and drained

1 onion, 1 half finely chopped (1/2 cup)

1 carrot, cut crosswise into thirds

1 celery stalk, cut crosswise into thirds

1 dried bay leaf

1 can (28 oz.) whole plum tomatoes, with juice

2 tbsp. extra-virgin olive oil, plus more for drizzling

2 garlic cloves, minced

1/8 tsp. red-pepper flakes

1 sprig rosemary

coarse salt and pepper, freshly ground

Directions:

Soak beans in water overnight. Drain, and transfer to a large pot. Cover beans with 4 inches water. Add the intact half of the onion, the carrot, celery, and bay leaf. Bring to a boil. Reduce heat and simmer until beans are tender but not bursting, about 1 hour. Drain and remove onion, carrot, celery, and bay leaf; discard. Pulse tomatoes, with juice, in a food processor until coarsely chopped. Heat oil in a medium heavy-bottomed pot over medium heat. Add chopped onion, the garlic, and red-pepper flakes. Cook, stirring occasionally, until onion and garlic are tender but not browned, about 3 minutes. Add tomatoes and rosemary. Bring to a boil. Add beans and simmer, stirring occasionally, until tomato sauce thickens, about 20 minutes. Season with salt and pepper. Serve warm and drizzle with oil just before serving.

112. Kimchi Fried Rice

Preparation time: 15 minutes

Servings: 4

Ingredients:

1 cup kimchi, cut into thumbnail size pieces

7 oz. pack enoki mushrooms, root removed (optional),

3 cups steamed white short/medium grain rice – if it is freshly cooked, leave it out for 5 to 10 mins at room temperature to cool down before cooking.

1/2 tsp. garlic, minced

1/4 cup kimchi juice (liquid from the bottom of the kimchi container)

1/2 tbsp. sesame oil

1/2 tbsp. cooking oil

1 to 2 tbsp. roasted sesame seeds, to garnish

(optional) 1/2 stalk green onion, thinly sliced

(optional) seaweed, roasted, seasoned, shredded

Directions:

On medium high heat preheat a pan/wok and once heated, add the cooking oil and spread it well with a spatula. Add the garlic, stir it fast for about 10 seconds. Add the kimchi and stir until 80% of it is cooked. Optionally, add the mushrooms and mix them well for a few seconds. Reduce the heat to medium-medium low. Add the rice and the kimchi juice. Mix everything together thoroughly. Add the sesame oil and mix well. Remove from heat. Garnish with sesame seeds, green onion and seaweed strips.

113. Biryani Rice

Preparation time: 25 minutes

Servings: 4

Ingredients:

2 cups basmati rice

3 cloves garlic crushed in a garlic press

1 tsp. ground cumin

1/2 tsp. ground turmeric

1/4 tsp. cayenne pepper or to taste

salt and freshly ground black pepper

3 tbsp. olive or canola oil

4 tsp. lemon juice

1/4 cup fresh cilantro or parsley, chopped

4 cardamom pods

2⅔ cups veggie stock

Directions:

Wash the rice in several changes of water and drain. Cover generously with fresh water and leave to soak for 30 minutes. Drain. Pour the oil into a heavy, medium pan and set over medium-high heat. Put the cardamom pods in the pan and sauté for about 10-15 seconds. Add garlic and sauté for another 10 seconds. Add veggie stock, bring to a boil. Add lemon juice, cumin, turmeric, cayenne, black pepper and salt. Add the drained rice and bring to a boil again. Cover tightly, turn heat to very, very low, and cook for about 25 minutes or until rice is soft.

114. Vegan Paella

Preparation time: 20 minutes

Servings: 4

Ingredients:

2½ cups vegetable stock

1/2 tsp. saffron threads

1½ tbsp. olive oil

1 large red onion, sliced

1 yellow bell pepper, sliced

1 red bell pepper, sliced

1 cup brown mushrooms, sliced

3 cloves garlic, minced

1 cup bomba rice

2 roma tomatoes, chopped

1½ tsp. paprika, smoked

salt and pepper, freshly ground, to taste

1 cup green peas

1 can artichoke hearts, drained and chopped

1/2 cup parsley, chopped

Directions:

Combine the stock and saffron threads in a medium saucepan and bring to the boil over high heat.

Reduce heat to low and maintain a simmer.

Meanwhile, heat paella pan on the stove with 1 - 1/2 tablespoons olive oil.

Add onion to paella pan and sauté for 2 minutes.

Add sliced red and yellow pepper and continue to sauté till softened, about 5 minutes.

Add the mushrooms and garlic and sauté for 5 minutes or until it has softened slightly.

Season liberally with salt and pepper. Increase heat to medium-high.

Add bomba rice, tomato and smoked paprika and cook, stirring, for 1 minute until well mixed through.

Reduce heat to medium-low.

Add one-third of the saffron infused stock and stir until just combined.

Let simmer uncovered for 5 minutes or until liquid is almost absorbed.

Add the next third of the stock and cook for 5 minutes uncovered or until almost absorbed.

Add remaining third of stock and cook for 5-10 minutes uncovered.

Sprinkle surface of paella with peas and artichoke hearts.

Cover entire pan in tin foil and leave to cook on a low heat for 12 minutes.

After 12 minutes, turn heat off but leave the paella pan covered with tin foil for another 10 minutes.

Remove tin foil after 10 minutes and garnish with parsley.

115. Rice with Fresh Vegetables

Preparation time: 20 minutes

Servings: 4

Ingredients:

2 tbsp. butter

1/2 cup orzo pasta or broken spaghetti

1 tbsp. extra-virgin olive oil

1 bunch asparagus, trimmed and chopped 1 carrot, cut into short matchsticks

2 shallots, chopped

2 cloves garlic, chopped

salt and pepper, freshly ground

2½ cups vegetable stock

1 cup long-grain white rice

1 tbsp. lemon zest, plus the juice of 1/2 lemon

1 tbsp. fresh thyme, chopped

1 bunch arugula, chopped

about 1 cup Parmigiano-Reggiano, grated

Directions: Melt the butter in a medium pot over medium-high heat. Add the pasta and cook until nutty and deep golden brown. Add the extra-virgin olive oil, 1 turn of the pan, then add the asparagus, carrot, shallots, garlic, salt and pepper. Cover and cook to sweat the vegetables, stirring occasionally, for 5 minutes. Stir in the stock, rice, lemon zest, thyme and browned pasta and bring to a boil. Cover the pot, lower the heat and simmer until the rice is just tender. Fold in the arugula, then stir in the lemon juice and cheese.

116. Eggplant Pasta

Preparation time: 15 minutes

Servings: 4

Ingredients:

1 pound large eggplant

1 tbsp. olive oil

1/4 tsp. garlic, minced

1/4 tsp. red pepper flakes

1 small tomato, seeded and chopped

3 tbsp. heavy cream

1 tbsp. basil, chiffonade

2 tbsp. parmesan cheese, grated

1 tbsp. breadcrumbs

1/4 cup pomegranate seeds

kosher salt

Directions:

Peel the eggplant, leaving 1 inch of skin at the top and bottom. Slice the eggplant lengthwise into 1/4-inch-thick slices. Place the eggplant slices on a cooling rack set over the sink and generously sprinkle with kosher salt. Wait 15 minutes, flip, sprinkle again, and wait another 15 minutes. Rinse thoroughly under cool water and gently squeeze out excess water. Place on paper towels and pat dry, then cut the slices into 1/4-inch-wide strips so that they resemble linguine. Heat a 10-inch sauté pan over medium-high heat and add the oil. When it shimmers, add the garlic and red pepper flakes and toss for 10 seconds. Add the eggplant and toss to coat. Add the tomato and toss for 15 to 20 seconds. Add the cream and toss for another 10 seconds. Finish with the basil and parmesan. Transfer to a serving dish, top with breadcrumbs. Sprinkle the pomegranate seeds, toss and serve immediately.

117. Stuffed Mushrooms

Preparation time: 30 minutes

Servings: 4

Ingredients:

8 small/medium size Portobello mushrooms

1 small stalk celery

2 cloves garlic, finely chopped

1/2 slice ginger, fresh

1 large onion, finely chopped

2 small red bell peppers, finely chopped

3 tbsp. pine nuts

4 tbsp. olive oil

2 tsp. soy sauce

salt and pepper and/or chili, to taste

Directions:

Cut and finely dice the stems of the mushrooms. Precook mushroom stems, ginger, garlic and pepper in the olive oil. Stir in all other ingredients into the vegetable mix after it is removed from heat. Oil the mushrooms and put them on the baking pan. Stuff the mushrooms, mounding them with the mix generously. Cook in an oven for 15-20 minutes until the top forms a crispy crust. Top the cooked mushrooms with some fresh herbs for a nice decor.

118. Fried Tomatoes

Preparation time: 25 minutes

Servings: 4

Ingredients:

8 ripe plum tomatoes, halved

2 tbsp. basil leaves, fresh chopped

1 tbsp. oregano, dry

1 tbsp. basil, dry

2 tbsp. rosemary, sprigs

2 cloves garlic, minced

3 tbsp. olive oil

salt and pepper, to taste

Directions:

Add some olive oil onto the frying pan, placing tomatoes cut-sides up. Sprinkle them with all herbs and garlic and drizzle with olive oil on top. Cover and cook on a lower heat at least for 5 minutes, then remove the cover and have them cooked until browned underneath. Top with some fresh greenery and serve immediately.

Chapter 6. Soups and Salads

119. Creamy Onion Soup

Preparation Time: 10minutes

Cooking Time: 65 minutes

Servings: 4

Ingredients:

3 tbsp olive oil

3 cups thinly sliced white onions

2 garlic cloves, thinly sliced

2 tsp almond flour

½ cup dry white wine

Salt and black pepper to taste

2 sprigs chopped thyme

2 cups hot vegetable broth

2 cups almond milk

1 cup grates Swiss cheese

Directions:

Heat the olive oil in a pot over medium heat. Sauté the onions for 10 minutes or until softened, stirring regularly to avoid browning. Reduce the heat to low and cook further for 15 minutes while occasionally stirring.

Mix in the garlic, cook further for 10 minutes or until the onions caramelize.

Stir in the almond flour well, wine, and increase the heat. Season with salt, black pepper, thyme, and pour in the hot vegetable broth. Cover the pot, bring to a boil, and then simmer for 30 minutes.

Pour in the almond milk and half of the Swiss cheese. Stir until the cheese melts, adjust the taste with salt, black pepper, and dish the soup.

Top with the remaining cheese and serve warm.

Nutrition:

Calories:183 , Total Fat:14.7g, Saturated Fat:7.6g, Total Carbs:8 g, Dietary Fiber2:g, Sugar: 2g, Protein:8 g, Sodium: 452mg

120. Lettuce and Cauliflower Soup

Preparation Time: 10 minutes

Cooking Time: 30 minutes

Servings: 4

Ingredients:

1 tbsp olive oil

2 tbsp butter

1 medium red onion, thinly sliced

3 garlic cloves, finely sliced

1 large head cauliflower, cut into florets

1 medium lettuce head, leaves extracted and chopped

4 cups vegetable stock

6 sprigs parsley, leaves extracted

Salt and black pepper to taste

1 tbsp fresh dill leaves for garnishing

1 cup grated provolone cheese for topping

Directions:

Heat the oil and butter in a large saucepan over medium heat and sauté the onion and garlic until softened and fragrant, 3 minutes.

Stir in the cauliflower, lettuce, and cook until the lettuce wilts, 3 minutes

Pour in the vegetable stock, parsley and season with salt and black pepper. Close the lid, bring to a boil, and then simmer until the cauliflower softens.

Open the lid and using an immersion blender, puree the soup until smooth. Adjust the taste with salt and black pepper.

Dish the soup, top with the provolone cheese, and serve warm.

Nutrition:

Calories: 312, Total Fat:21g, Saturated Fat:11.9g, Total Carbs: 15g, Dietary Fiber:5g, Sugar: 6g, Protein: 19g, Sodium: 63mg

121. Spring Vegetable Soup

Preparation Time: 8 minutes

Cooking Time: 13 minutes

Servings: 4

Ingredients:

4 cups vegetable stock

3 cups green beans, chopped

2 cups asparagus, chopped

1 cup pearl onions, peeled and halved

2 cups baby spinach

1 tbsp garlic powder

Salt and white pepper to taste

2 cups grated cheddar cheese for topping

Directions:

In a large pot, add the vegetable stock, green beans, asparagus, and pearl onions. Bring to a boil over medium heat and then simmer until the vegetables soften, 10 minutes.

Stir in the spinach, allow slight wilting, and adjust the taste with salt and white pepper.

Dish the soup, top with the cheddar cheese, and serve warm.

Nutrition:

Calories:405 , Total Fat:32.2g, Saturated Fat:5.2g, Total Carbs: 18g, Dietary Fiber:4g, Sugar: 9g, Protein: 16g, Sodium: 64mg

122. Creamy Garlicky Tofu Soup

Preparation Time: 10 minutes

Cooking Time: 11 minutes

Servings: 4

Ingredients:

1 tbsp olive oil

1 large white onion, finely chopped

3 tbsp minced garlic

1 tsp ginger puree

1 cup vegetable stock

2 parsnips, peeled and chopped

Salt and black pepper to taste

2 (14 oz) silken tofu, drained and rinsed

2 cups almond milk

1 tbsp chopped fresh basil

1 tbsp chopped fresh parsley to garnish

Chopped toasted pecans for topping

Directions:

Heat the olive oil in a saucepan and sauté the onion, garlic, and ginger puree until fragrant and soft, 3 minutes

Mix in the vegetable stock, parsnips, salt, and black pepper. Cover and cook until the parsnips soften, 6 minutes.

Add the silken tofu and immediately puree the soup using an immersion blender until very smooth.

Stir in the almond milk, basil, and cook further for 2 minutes with frequent stirring to prevent the tofu from curdling.

Dish the soup, garnish with the parsley, pecans, and serve warm.

Nutrition:

Calories:171 , Total Fat:13.9g, Saturated Fat:3.4g, Total Carbs: 12g, Dietary Fiber:6g, Sugar: 4g, Protein: 3g, Sodium: 35mg

123. Kale Ginger Soup with Avocados

Preparation Time: 8 minutes

Cooking Time: 8 minutes

Servings: 4

Ingredients:

1 tbsp butter

1 tbsp sesame oil + extra for drizzling

1 small onion, finely sliced

3 garlic cloves, minced

2 tsp ginger paste

2 cups baby kale, chopped

2 cups chopped green beans

4 cups vegetable stock

3 tbsp chopped fresh cilantro + extra for garnish

Salt and black pepper to taste

1 large avocado, pitted, peeled, and diced for topping

Directions:

Heat the butter and sesame oil in a large pot over medium heat.

Sauté the onions, garlic, and garlic until softened and fragrant, 3 minutes.

Mix in the kale, green beans, vegetable stock, and cilantro. Season with salt, black pepper, and cook covered until the vegetables soften, 5 minutes.

Open the lid, adjust the taste with salt, black pepper, and dish the soup.

Top with the avocado and serve warm.

Nutrition:

Calories:212 , Total Fat:16.1g, Saturated Fat:8.6g, Total Carbs: 14g, Dietary Fiber:2g, Sugar:5 g, Protein:5 g, Sodium: 124mg

124. Creamy Tomato & Turnip Soup

Preparation Time: 10 minutes

Cooking Time: 18 minutes

Servings: 4

Ingredients:

2 tbsp butter

1 large red onion, chopped

4 garlic cloves, minced

6 red bell peppers, deseeded and sliced

2 turnips, peeled and diced

3 cups chopped tomatoes

4 cups vegetable stock

Salt and black pepper to taste

1 cup heavy cream

½ cup grated Swiss cheese

2 cups toasted chopped cashew nuts

Directions:

Melt the butter in a large pot over medium heat and sauté the onion and garlic until softened and fragrant, 3 minutes.

Stir in the bell peppers, turnips, tomatoes, vegetable stock, and season with salt and black pepper.

Bring to a boil and then simmer until the turnips and very tender, 15 minutes.

Insert an immersion blender and puree the soup until smooth.

Mix in the heavy cream and adjust the taste with salt and black pepper.

Dish the soup, top with the Swiss cheese, cashew nuts, and serve warm.

Nutrition:

Calories: 486, Total Fat:41.3g, Saturated Fat:14.5g, Total Carbs:14 g, Dietary Fiber:2g, Sugar:8 g, Protein: 17g, Sodium:601 mg

125. Italian Cheese Soup

Preparation Time: 12 minutes

Cooking Time: 20 minutes

Servings: 4

Ingredients:

1 tbsp avocado oil

6 slices vegan bacon, chopped

4 tbsp butter

1 small white onion, roughly chopped

3 garlic cloves, minced

2 tbsp chopped fresh Italian mixed herbs

2 cups peeled and cubed rutabagas

3 ½ cups vegetable broth

Salt and black pepper to taste

1 cup almond milk

1 cup grated provolone

2 tbsp chopped scallions for garnishing

Directions:

Heat the olive oil in a medium pot over medium heat and cook the vegan bacon until brown and crispy, 5 minutes. Transfer to a plate and set aside.

Melt the butter in the pot and sauté the onion, garlic, and mixed herbs until fragrant, 3 minutes.

Stir in the rutabagas, season with salt, black pepper, and cook for 10 to 12 minutes or until the rutabagas soften.

Open the lid, insert an immersion blender, and process the soup until very smooth.

Stir in the almond milk and provolone cheese until the cheese melts.

Adjust the taste with salt, black pepper, and dish the soup into serving bowls.

Garnish with the scallions and serve warm.

Nutrition:

Calories:646 , Total Fat:63.7g, Saturated Fat:40.1g, Total Carbs:24 g, Dietary Fiber:13g, Sugar: 2g, Protein: 8g, Sodium:16 mg

126. Chilled Lemongrass and Avocado Soup

Preparation Time: 5 minutes

Cooking Time: 5 minutes

Servings: 4

Ingredients:

4 cups chopped avocado pulp

2 stalks lemongrass, chopped

4 cups vegetable broth

2 lemons, juiced

3 tbsp chopped mint + extra to garnish

Salt and black pepper to taste

2 cups coconut cream

Directions:

Over low heat, bring the avocado, lemongrass, and vegetable broth to a slow boil until the avocado warms through, 3 to 5 minutes.

Add the remaining Ingredients and process until smooth using an immersion blender.

Adjust the taste with salt, black pepper, and dish the soup.

Nutrition:

Calories:391 , Total Fat:37.3g, Saturated Fat:28.3g, Total Carbs: 13g, Dietary Fiber5:g, Sugar:3 g, Protein:7 g, Sodium:68 mg

127. Mixed Mushroom Soup

Preparation Time: 10minutes

Cooking Time: 29minutes

Servings: 4

Ingredients:

4 oz unsalted butter

1 small onion, finely chopped

1 clove garlic, minced

5 oz. white button mushrooms, chopped

5 oz. cremini mushrooms, chopped

5 oz. oyster mushrooms, chopped

½ lb celery root, chopped

½ tsp dried rosemary

3 cups vegetable broth

1 tbsp plain vinegar

1 cup cashew cream

4 basil leaves, chopped

2 tbsp chopped blanched almonds

Directions:

Melt the butter in a medium pot and sauté the Ingredients up to the vegetable stock until softened, 5 minutes.

Mix in the vegetable broth, vinegar, and bring the food to a boil. Reduce the heat to low and simmer until the liquid reduces by one-third.

Mix in the cashew cream and puree the Ingredients using an immersion blender. Simmer for 2 minutes.

Dish the soup, garnish with the basil, almonds, and serve warm.

Nutrition:

Calories: 325, Total Fat:30.6g, Saturated Fat:14.2g, Total Carbs:11 g, Dietary Fiber:2g, Sugar: 3g, Protein: g, Sodium: 398mg

128. Coconut Pumpkin Soup

Preparation Time: 8 minutes

Cooking Time: 15 minutes

Servings: 4

Ingredients:

2 tbsp + 2 tbsp butter

2 small red onions

2 garlic cloves

1 cup chopped pumpkins

2 cups vegetable broth

Salt and black pepper to taste

½ cup coconut cream

½ lemon, juiced

¾ cup mayonnaise

Pumpkin seeds for garnishing

Directions:

Melt 2 tbsp of butter in a medium pot and sauté the onion and garlic until softened and fragrant, 3 minutes.

Stir in the pumpkins, vegetable broth, salt, and black pepper. Close the lid, allow boiling, and then simmer for 10 minutes

Open the lid, add the remaining butter, coconut cream, and puree the soup with an immersion blender until smooth.

Mix in the lemon juice, mayonnaise, and adjust the taste with salt and black pepper.

Dish the soup, garnish with the pumpkin seeds, and serve warm.

Nutrition:

Calories:566 , Total Fat:57.7g, Saturated Fat:43.5g, Total Carbs:15 g, Dietary Fiber:7g, Sugar: 1g, Protein:6g, Sodium: 87mg

129. Mixed Green Soup

Preparation Time: 6minutes

Cooking Time: 10minutes

Servings: 4

Ingredients:

3 tbsp butter

1 cup fresh spinach, coarsely chopped

1 cup fresh kale, coarsely chopped

½ cup mustard greens, coarsely chopped

1 large avocado, pitted and peeled

3 ½ cups coconut cream

1 cup vegetable broth

1 tsp onion powder

1 tsp garlic powder

3 tbsp chopped fresh mint leaves

Salt and black pepper to taste

1 lime, juiced

Directions:

Melt the butter in a medium pot and sauté the greens until wilted. Add the avocado, coconut cream, vegetable broth, onion powder, garlic powder, mint leaves, salt, and black pepper. Simmer for 10 minutes or until the avocado warms through.

Insert an immersion blender and puree until smooth.

Mix in the lime juice, adjust the taste with salt, black pepper, and dish the soup.

Nutrition:

Calories:401 , Total Fat:41.2g, Saturated Fat:g28.9, Total Carbs:9 g, Dietary Fiber:3g, Sugar: 3g, Protein:3 g, Sodium: 271mg

130. Celery Dill Soup

Preparation Time: 5minutes

Cooking Time: 21 minutes

Servings: 4

Ingredients:

2 tbsp coconut oil

1 cup chopped celery

1 medium white onion

1 garlic clove

¼ cup fresh dill, roughly chopped

1 tsp cumin powder

¼ tsp nutmeg powder

1 small head cauliflower, cut into florets

3½ cups seasoned vegetable stock

5 oz. butter

1 lemon, juiced

¼ cup coconut cream

Salt and black pepper

Directions:

Heat the avocado oil over in a medium pot over medium heat and sauté the celery, onion, and garlic until fragrant and soft, about 5 minutes.

Stir in the following Ingredients up to the butter, cover the lid, and cook over low heat for 10 minutes or until the cauliflower softens.

Puree the soup with an immersion blender until very smooth and mix in the butter, lemon juice, coconut cream, and adjust the taste with salt and black pepper.

Dish the soup and serve warm.

Nutrition:

Calories:340 , Total Fat:g30, Saturated Fat:13.2g, Total Carbs: 15g, Dietary Fiber:2g, Sugar: 8g, Protein:3g, Sodium:165 mg

131. Broccoli Squash Soup

Preparation Time: 5 minutes

Cooking Time : 20 minutes

Servings : 4

Ingredients:

1 large yellow squash, peeled and cubed

10 oz. broccoli, cut into florets

3 cups vegetable stock

Salt and black pepper to taste

1 garlic clove, minced

1 cup cashew cream

3 oz. butter

½ cup chopped fresh oregano

Directions:

Put the squash and broccoli into a pot and cover with the vegetable stock. Bring the Ingredients to a boil over medium heat until the vegetables are soft, about 10 minutes.

Season with salt, black pepper and add the garlic. Simmer the soup for 10 minutes or until the broccoli softens.

Add the remaining Ingredients and puree using an immersion blender until very smooth.

Adjust the taste with salt and black pepper, and dish the soup.

Serve warm.

Nutrition:

Calories:339 , Total Fat:g29.6, Saturated Fat:16.2g, Total Carbs: 12g, Dietary Fiber:3g, Sugar: 4g, Protein: 11g, Sodium: 214mg

132. Tofu Goulash Soup

Preparation Time: 10 minutes

Cooking Time: 28 minutes

Servings: 4

Ingredients:

4¼ oz butter

1 ½ cup extra firm tofu, pressed and crumbled

1 white onion

2 garlic cloves

8 oz yellow squash, chopped

1 red bell pepper, deseeded and diced

1 tbsp paprika powder

¼ tsp red chili flakes

1 tbsp dried basil

½ tbsp crushed cardamom seeds

Salt and black pepper to taste

1 ½ cups crushed tomatoes

3 cups vegetable broth

1½ tsp red wine vinegar

Chopped cilantro to serve

Directions:

Melt the butter in a medium pot over medium heat and sauté the onion and garlic for 3 minutes or until fragrant and softened.

Stir in the tofu and cook until brown, 5 minutes.

Add the remaining Ingredients up to the red wine vinegar, cover the lid, bring to a boil, and then simmer for 10 to 15 minutes.

Open the lid, mix in the red wine and adjust the taste with salt and black pepper.

Dish the soup, garnish with the cilantro, and serve warm.

Nutrition:

Calories:257 , Total Fat:25g, Saturated Fat:5.4g, Total Carbs:4 g, Dietary Fiber:2g, Sugar:1 g, Protein:5 g, Sodium: 520mg

133. Cauliflower Soup

Preparation Time: 10 Minutes

Cooking Time: 20 Minutes

Servings: 2)

Ingredients

5 cups vegetable broth or water

1 medium onion chopped

1 - 2 stalks leek thinly sliced

2 cloves garlic crushed

1 lb. cauliflower cut in big chunks

1 teaspoon salt

1/2 teaspoon pepper

1 teaspoon fresh basil

1/4 cup almond flour

2/3 cup Water

1 cup grated goat cheese

1/2 cup milk

Instructions

Add the first 8 Ingredients (including basil) to the instant pot and close the lid. Make sure the valve is set to Seal and press Pressure cook (or Manual). Set the time with the + /- buttons for 5 minutes.

While cooking, stir in flour and water until smooth. When the IP beeps, flip the valve from Sealing to Venting and when the pin drops, press Cancel and remove the lid.

Press the Sauté button and cook again, stirring frequently. Whisk the flour-water mixture and add about half of it to the soup.

Use a hand blender to puree the soup. Or use a blender or food processor and put it back in the pan.

Press Cancel and add the chees. Stir until melted. DO NOT cook after the cheese has gone in. Add the milk. Try to add salt and pepper to your taste. Serve with a pinch of grated cheese.

Nutrition:

Calories 202, Total Fat 8.4g, Saturated Fat 4.4g, Cholesterol 20mg , Sodium 1345mg, Total Carbohydrate 23.2g , Dietary Fiber 7.8g , Total Sugars 11.3g, Protein 12.6g

134. Pumpkin Soup

Preparation Time: 10 Minutes

Cooking Time: 20 Minutes

Servings: 2)

Ingredients

1lb pumpkin peeled, and seeded 1/2-1-inch cubes

1 cup vegetable broth or water

1 teaspoon dried rosemary

1/4 teaspoon grated cinnamon

1/2 teaspoon salt

1 cup coconut milk

2 tablespoons butter

1 tablespoon almond flour

Instructions

Mix the pumpkin cubes, broth, rosemary, cinnamon, and salt in an Instant Pot. Lock the lid onto the pot.

Press Soup/Broth, Pressure Cook or Manual on High pressure for 5 minutes with the Keep Warm setting off. The valve must be closed.

Use the quick release method to return the pot pressure to normal. Unlock the lid and open the pot. Add coconut milk.

Use an immersion blender to puree the soup right in the pot. Or work in halves to puree the soup in a covered blender. If necessary, pour all the soup back into the pan.

Press the SAUTÉ button and set it for LOW, LESS, or CUSTOM 250°F. Set the timer for 5 minutes.

Bring the soup to a simmer, stirring often. In the meantime, place the butter in a small bowl or measuring container and place in the microwave in 5-second increments. Use a fork to mix the flour and make a thin paste.

When the soup is boiling, Whisk the butter mixture in the pan. Continue whisking until the soup is a bit thick, about 1 minute. Turn off the SAUTÉ function and allow it to cool for a few minutes before serving.

Nutrition:

Calories 415, Total Fat 41g, Saturated Fat 32.9g, Cholesterol 31mg , Sodium 1064mg, Total Carbohydrate 11.5g, Dietary Fiber 3.3g, Total Sugars 5.2g, Protein 5.9g

135. Vegetarian Spinach Soup

Preparation Time: 15 Minutes

Cooking Time: 20 Minutes

Servings: 2

Ingredients

½ tablespoon coconut oil

¼ onion, finely chopped

½ stalk leek, finely chopped

1 teaspoon garlic powder

1 teaspoon basil, freshly chopped

¼ teaspoon red pepper flakes (optional)

Salt

Freshly ground black pepper

2 cups vegetable broth

1 (15.5-oz.) can chickpea, drained and rinsed

Juice of 1 lemon

1 large bunch Spinach, removed from stems and torn into medium pieces

Instructions

In an instant pot press the SAUTÉ button and set it for Medium, heat oil. Add onion, leek and cook until slightly soft, 6 minutes. Add garlic powder, basil, and red pepper flakes and cook until fragrant, 1 minute more. Season with salt and pepper.

Add broth, water, and chickpea and Spinach. Press Soup/Broth, Pressure Cook or Manual on High pressure for 10 minutes with the Keep Warm setting off. The valve must be closed.

Use the quick release method to return the pot pressure to normal. Unlock the lid and open the pot.

Use an immersion blender to puree the soup right in the pot.

Press the SAUTÉ button and set it for LOW, 250°F. Set the timer for 5 minutes.

Bring the soup to a simmer, stirring often.

Serve.

Nutrition:

Calories 336, Total Fat 7.8g, Saturated Fat 2.7g, Cholesterol 0mg , Sodium 669mg, Total Carbohydrate 50.7g, Dietary Fiber 15.2g, Total Sugars 9.8g, Protein 20.1g

136. Green Soup

Preparation Time: 10 Minutes

Cooking Time: 35 Minutes

Servings: 2

Ingredients

1 small onion cut into 3/4-inch pieces

1/3 cup rice

1 tablespoon vegetable oil

1 teaspoon garlic powder

Salt

1/4 cup Greek yogurt

1 tsp minced fresh mint

1/4 tsp finely grated lime zest plus 1/2 tsp juice

6 Oz. Collard Greens stemmed and chopped

4 Oz Spinach stemmed and chopped

1 cup Beet Greens

Instructions

Add broth, onion, rice, oil, garlic powder, and 1/2 teaspoon salt to blender. Lock lid in place, then select Soup program 2 (for creamy soups).

In the meantime, combine Greek yogurt, mint, lime zest and juice, and remaining 1/4 teaspoon salt in bowl; refrigerate until ready to serve.

Pause program 12 minutes before it has completed. Carefully remove lid and stir in Collard Greens and Spinach until completely submerged.

Return lid and resume program. Pause program 1 minute before it has completed. Stir in beet greens. Return lid and resume program. Once program has completed, adjust soup consistency with extra broth as needed and season with salt and pepper to taste. Drizzle individual portions with yogurt sauce before serving.

Nutrition:

Calories 306, Total Fat 9.7g, Saturated Fat 1.8g, Cholesterol 1mg 0%, Sodium 225mg, Total Carbohydrate 48.7g, Dietary Fiber 12.6g , Total Sugars 3.4g, Protein 13.6g

137. Tofu and Quinoa Soup

Preparation Time: 10 Minutes

Cooking Time: 40 Minutes

Servings: 2

Ingredients

4 ounces mushrooms trimmed and quartered

1 small onion cut into 3/4-inch pieces

1 1/2 tablespoons tomato paste

1 tablespoon olive oil

1 teaspoon garlic powder

1 teaspoon minced fresh basil

1/4 teaspoon pepper

3 cups vegetable broth

1 carrot peeled and cut into 3/4-inch pieces

2 Oz tofu and cut into ¼-inch pieces

1/4 cup quinoa

2 tablespoons minced fresh coriander

Instructions

Microwave mushrooms, onion, tomato paste, oil, garlic powder , basil, and pepper in Instant pot, stirring occasionally, until vegetables are softened, about 5 minutes; transfer to blender along with broth, carrot. Lock lid in place, then select Soup Program.

Pause program once preheating ends. Carefully remove lid and stir in tofu and quinoa. Return lid and resume program. Once program has completed, season with salt and pepper to taste. Sprinkle individual portions with coriander and serve.

Nutrition:

Calories 236, Total Fat 12.2g, Saturated Fat 1.9g,Cholesterol 0mg, , Sodium 1188mg, Total Carbohydrate 18.6g, Dietary Fiber 3.5g, , Total Sugars 6.7g, Protein 15.3g

138. Barley Vegetable Soup

Preparation Time: 10 Minutes

Cooking Time: 30 Minutes

Servings: 2

Ingredients

1 tablespoon butter

1 medium onion, chopped

1 carrot, peeled and cut into thin rounds

1 teaspoon garlic powder

½ large zucchini, cut into 1/2" pieces

1 (14.5-oz.) can diced tomatoes

1 cup Kidney beans

½ cup barley

¼ teaspoon. ground cumin

4 cups vegetable broth

4 oz. kale, ribs removed and leaves thinly sliced

½ tablespoon fresh lemon juice

Crushed red pepper flakes, for serving

Instructions

Soak the beans. In a large bowl, cover the kidney beans with 2 to 3 inches of cold water. Soak at room temperature for 8 hours, or overnight. Drain and rinse.

Pressure cook the beans and barley. Pour 3 cups of water into the inner pot of Instant pot,. Lock the lid into place. Select Pressure Cook or Manual, and adjust the pressure to High and the time to 8 minutes. Make sure the steam release knob is in the sealed position. After cooking, naturally release the pressure for 5 minutes, then quick release any remaining pressure. Unlock and remove the lid, Drain the beans and barley, reserving 1 cup of bean and barley water. Wipe the inner pot dry.

Sauté the vegetables. Select Sauté, and pour in the oil. Once hot, add the onion and garlic powder and cook for 2 minutes. Add the zucchini, carrot, kale, and Sauté for 1 minute. Add the salt, 1 tsp of, and pepper. Stir to combine. Add the 1 cup of bean barley water and the vegetable broth.

Pressure cook the vegetables and beans and barley. Lock the lid into place. Select Soup, and adjust the pressure to High and the time to 20 minutes. Make sure the steam release knob is in the sealed position. After cooking, naturally release the pressure. Unlock and remove the lid.

Finish the soup. Unlock and remove the lid. Stir in the remaining and serve hot.

Nutrition:

Calories 373, Total Fat 8.1g, Saturated Fat 2.7g, Cholesterol 8mg , Sodium 828mg, Total Carbohydrate 58.2g, Dietary Fiber 15g , Total Sugars 9.7g, Protein 19.6g

139. Cabbage Soup

Preparation Time: 10 Minutes

Cooking Time: 20 Minutes

Servings: 2

Ingredients

1 head cabbage

½ tablespoon dried basil

2 Oz Cheddar cheese chunks

½ tablespoon coconut cream

½ teaspoon garlic powder

Salt

Instructions

Add all Ingredients to the blender pitcher and secure lid.

Select "Soup 1" setting for 20:00 minutes.

Garnish with shredded cheddar cheese and serve.

Nutrition:

Calories 213, Total Fat 10.5g, Saturated Fat 6.8g, Cholesterol 29mg , Sodium 316mg, Total Carbohydrate 21.8g, Dietary Fiber 9.1g , Total Sugars 11.9g, Protein 11.8g

140. Almond Broccoli Soup

Preparation Time: 05 Minutes

Cooking Time: 20 Minutes

Servings: 2

Ingredients

1/2 cup roasted Almond divided

2 1/2 cups Vegetable broth divided

½ tablespoon fresh basil leaves chopped

½ tablespoon fresh oregano leaves chopped

1 teaspoon garlic powder

15 Oz can chickpeas drained and rinsed

1 small onion roughly chopped

1 small head broccoli cut into florets

Instructions

Add almond to the blender pitcher and secure the lid.

Touch PULSE, then touch START.

When the Pulse program is complete, scrape down the sides and bottom of the pitcher.

Add 1/2 cup broth and secure the lid.

Touch PULSE, then START.

When the Pulse program is complete, add the remaining broth, herbs, garlic powder, chickpeas, onion and broccoli--in that order-- and secure the lid.

Touch SOUP two times and use +/- to set the time to 14 minutes, then touch START.

Adjust seasonings and Serve.

Nutrition:

Calories192, Total Fat 9.7g, Saturated Fat 0.7g, Cholesterol 0mg, Sodium 450mg, Total Carbohydrate 20.4g, Dietary Fiber 4g, Total Sugars 6.4g, Protein 7.8g

141. Jackfruit Stew

Preparation Time: 10 Minutes

Cooking Time: 25 Minutes

Servings: 2

Ingredients

1 large onion chopped

3 cloves garlic minced

1 1/2 cup vegetable broth

1 teaspoon salt

1/2 teaspoon pepper

1 cup jackfruit

1 sweet potatoes cut into 1 inch pieces

1 zucchini cut into 1 inch pieces

½ cup frozen peas

1 tablespoon corn-starch

3 tablespoons Water

2 tablespoons chopped fresh parsley

Instructions

Mix the first five Ingredients, including the jackfruit, in the instant pot. Close the lid and make sure the valve is set to Sealing. Push Pressure Cook (or Manual) and use the +/− button to get to 20 minutes.

During cooking, cut sweet potatoes and carrots with or without peel into 1-inch pieces. Make a mixture by stirring the corn-starch in the water until smooth.

When the Instant pot beeps, let it go for 10 minutes. Natural release the remaining pressure and open the pot when the pin drops.

Add the sweet potatoes and carrots (not the peas) and gently squeeze them into the liquid. Close the lid and press hit pressure (or manual). Set the cooking time to 4 minutes. When it's done, take a quick release (pin drop), open the pot.

Tap Cancel then sauté. Stir in the corn-starch and add about half of the mortar as the stew cooks. Boil to thicken it, and if you want thicker, add more.

Press Cancel and add frozen peas. The heat of the stew is enough to cook them without turning them into mush. Add salt and pepper if necessary. Add the parsley if you use it,

Nutrition:

Calories 267, Total Fat 1.8g, Saturated Fat 0.4g, Cholesterol 0mg , Sodium 1786mg, Total Carbohydrate 56g, Dietary Fiber 8.1g, Total Sugars 7.5g, Protein 10g

142. Ginger & Turmeric Carrot Soup

Preparation Time: 10 Minutes

Cooking Time: 25 Minutes

Servings: 2

Ingredients

½ tablespoon butter

1 onion and sliced

1-1/2   cups chopped carrots

½ cup chopped pumpkin

¼ cup tomato, chopped

1 teaspoon garlic powder

1 tablespoon grated ginger

1 tablespoon turmeric powder

Salt & pepper to taste

3 cups vegetable broth

1 cup coconut milk

Instructions

Set on SAUTE mode and pour in the butter.

Add in the diced onion, carrots, and mix until combined.

Sauté for a few minutes or until the vegetables become soft, about 5 minutes.

Stir in the garlic powder, ginger and turmeric powder.

Add in the pumpkin, tomatoes, broth, coconut milk and stirring to combine.

Lock the lid in place and close the stem vent.

Set on MANUAL or PRESSURE COOK on HIGH PRESSURE for 4 minutes.

Allow the Instant Pot to natural release for 5 minutes once timer goes off.

Remove lid and stir to combine.

Enjoy!

Nutrition:

Calories 435, Total Fat 34.3g, Saturated Fat 28g, Cholesterol 8mg , Sodium 1228mg, Total Carbohydrate 25.1g, Dietary Fiber 7.4g , Total Sugars 11.2g, Protein 12.2g

143. Coconut Tofu Soup

Preparation Time: 10 Minutes

Cooking Time: 10 Minutes

Servings: 2

Ingredients

2 cups vegetable broth or water

1/2 pound tofu

½ cup full fat coconut milk

1 tablespoon ginger

2 whole red chills

½ tablespoon lemon zest

1 teaspoon maple syrup

1/2 teaspoon salt

1/4 cup fresh lime juice from 2 or 3 limes

Chopped fresh parsley for garnish

Lime wedges for serving

Instructions

In the Instant Pot, combine the broth, tofu, half the coconut milk, the ginger, chills (if using) lemon zest, maple syrup, and salt.

Secure the lid on theInstant pot. Close the pressure-release valve. Select MANUAL or PRESSURE COOK and set the pot at LOW pressure for 1 minute. At the end of the cooking time, quick release the pressure.

Stir in the remaining coconut milk, and lime juice.

Divide the soup among two serving bowls. Garnish with parsley and serve with lime wedges alongside for squeezing.

Nutrition:

Calories 238, Total Fat 19.2g, Saturated Fat 13.7g, Cholesterol 0mg , Sodium 31mg, Total Carbohydrate 10.3g, Dietary Fiber 2.9g , Total Sugars 5g, Protein 11g

144. Millet Soup

Preparation Time: 10 Minutes

Cooking Time: 30 Minutes

Servings: 2

Ingredients

½ tablespoon butter

1/4 cup Onion

½ cup chopped Parsnips,

½ cup sliced leeks,

1 teaspoon garlic powder

½ tablespoon lemon zest

Pinch of salt & pepper

¼ cup millet

2 cups vegetable broth

½ cup soy milk

1/8 cup lemon juice

1 cup fresh Swiss chard

Instructions

Heat the butter in an Instant pot and select SAUTE function. When butter melts add the onion, parsnips, leeks, and garlic powder and sauté until soft, about 5 minutes.

Add broth and millet, salt and pepper and stir to combine. Close the lid and make sure the valve is set to Sealing. Push Pressure Cook (or Manual) and use the +/− button to get to 20 minutes.

When the Instant pot beeps, let it go for 10 minutes. Natural release the remaining pressure and open the pot when the pin drops.

Once the Millet is cooked and soft, stir in the soy milk, lemon juice, and Swiss chard. Stir until Swiss chard is wilted.

Close the lid and press hit pressure (or manual). Set the cooking time to 4 minutes. When it's done, take a quick release (pin drop), open the Instant pot.

Serve immediately and enjoy! Soup can be frozen and reheated as desired.

Nutrition:

Calories 249, Total Fat 6.8g, Saturated Fat 2.7g, Cholesterol 8mg , Sodium 867mg, Total Carbohydrate 35.8g, Dietary Fiber 5.4g , Total Sugars 7.2g, Protein 11.3g

145. White lima beans Stew

Preparation Time: 15 Minutes

Cooking Time: 40 Minutes

Servings: 2

Ingredients

½ cup kale

 ½ tablespoons coconut oil

1 medium onion, chopped

½ teaspoon ginger powder

 ½ small bell pepper, seeded and finely chopped

½ teaspoon garlic powder

¼ tablespoon curry powder

1 medium zucchini, peeled and thinly sliced

¼ medium head broccoli, broken into bite-size florets

½ (15 ounce) can white lima beans, rinsed

1 small diced tomato

¼ cup almond milk

2 cups vegetable broth or water

Instructions

In a large bowl, add the white lima beans and soak at room temperature for 8 to 24 hours. Drain and rinse.

Select Sauté and adjust to Normal or Medium heat. Add the coconut oil to the inner pot of Instant pot and heat. Add the onion and zucchini and sprinkle with 1/4 teaspoon of salt. Cook, stirring often, until the onion pieces separate and soften. Add the garlic powder and ginger powder cook for about 1 minute, or until fragrant. Add the drained white lima beans, remaining 1/4 teaspoon of salt tomatoes and broth.

Lock the lid into place. Select Pressure Cook or Manual, and adjust the pressure to High and the time to 12 minutes. After cooking, let the pressure release naturally for 10 minutes, then quick release any remaining pressure.

Unlock the lid. Stir in the broccoli, kale and bell pepper and almond milk bring to a simmer to heat it through and thicken the sauce slightly.

Serve.

Nutrition:

Calories 205, Total Fat 11.4g, Saturated Fat 9.4g, Cholesterol 0mg , Sodium 121mg, Total Carbohydrate 23.4g, Dietary Fiber 6.3g, Total Sugars 8.4g, Protein 6.3g

146. Lentil Soup with Spinach

Preparation Time: 10 Minutes

Cooking Time: 40 Minutes

Servings: 2

Ingredients

¼ cup lentils

4 cups water, divided

1 tablespoon butter

1 small onion, diced

1 small beetroot, diced

½ teaspoon salt, divided

1/8 teaspoon ground pepper

½ teaspoon garlic powder,

¼ teaspoon ground coriander

½ cup chopped spinach

1 tablespoon chopped fresh parsley

½ cup small sweet potatoes, quartered

Juice of 1 lime, plus wedges for serving

Instructions

Wash the lentils very well and pick out any stones.

Add lentils and water to the Instant Pot and stir well.

Cover the Instant Pot and lock it in.

Make sure the vent on top is set to "sealing". Set manual or pressure cook timer for 25 minutes.

Once timer reaches zero, quick release the pressure. Keep aside

Then Select Sauté and adjust to Medium heat. Add the butter to the Instant pot and heat until melt. Add the onions and beetroot, sweet potato, and sprinkle salt and pepper. Cook, stirring often, until the onion soften. Add the garlic powder and grounded coriander cook for about 1 minute, or until fragrant. Add water and Lock the lid into place. Select Pressure Cook or Manual, and adjust the pressure to High and the time to 5 minutes. After cooking, let the pressure release naturally for 5minutes, then quick release any remaining pressure.

Unlock the lid. Stir in the spinach and bring to a simmer to heat it through spinach wilt. Then add cooked lentils and adjust it tasty to add salt and pepper.

Serve and enjoy.

Nutrition:

Calories 211, Total Fat 6.2g, Saturated Fat 3.7g, Cholesterol 15mg , Sodium 689mg, Total Carbohydrate 31.7g, Dietary Fiber 9.4g , Total Sugars 6.2g, Protein 8.4g

147. Chickpea and Mushroom Soup

Preparation Time: 05 Minutes

Cooking Time: 30 Minutes

Servings: 2

Ingredients

½ tablespoon avocado oil

8 ounces mushrooms sliced/chopped

¼ onion chopped

½ teaspoon garlic powder

½ (15 Oz) can chickpeas, drained & rinsed

2 cups vegetable broth

½ tablespoon dried Italian seasoning

½ teaspoon dried basil

Pinch of hot pepper flakes

Salt & pepper to taste

Instructions

Select Sauté and adjust to NORMAL heat. Add the avocado oil to the Instant pot and heat. Add garlic powder and onion and cook until the onions are slightly opaque and beginning to brown Add mushrooms. As the mushrooms start to soften, add the spices and the chickpeas. Season with salt and pepper .Add broth and Lock the lid into place. Select Pressure Cook or Manual, and adjust the pressure to High and the time to 20minutes. After cooking, let the pressure release naturally for 5minutes, then quick release any remaining pressure. Unlock the lid.

Adjust the seasoning and serve.

Nutrition:

Calories163, Total Fat 4g, Cholesterol 2mg, Sodium 955mg, Total Carbohydrate 21.5g, Dietary Fiber 4.6g , Total Sugars 4.2g, Protein 12.6g

148. Corn Potato Stew

Preparation Time: 10 Minutes

Cooking Time: 25 Minutes

Servings: 2

Ingredients

1 cup vegetable broth

1 cup water

½ pounds potatoes, peeled, and cut into 2-inch pieces

1 medium onion

¼ teaspoon garlic powder,

½ teaspoons dried basil, crushed

½ teaspoon chili powder

½ teaspoon ground cumin

¼ teaspoon salt

1 cup sweet corns, rinsed and drained

½ cup pinto beans, rinsed and drained

½ tablespoon fresh cilantro

Instructions

Add all of the Ingredients to the Instant Pot and stir well.

Cover the Instant Pot and lock it in.

Lock the lid in place and close the stem vent.

Set on MANUAL or PRESSURE COOK on HIGH PRESSURE for 20 minutes.

Allow the IP to natural release for 5 minutes once timer goes off.

Remove lid and stir to combine.

Enjoy!

Nutrition:

Calories358, Total Fat 2.6g, Saturated Fat 0.5g ,Cholesterol 0mg, , Sodium 710mg, Total Carbohydrate 69g , Dietary Fiber 13.8g, , Total Sugars 7.7g, Protein 18g

149. Tempeh wild rice Soup

Preparation Time: 05 Minutes

Cooking Time: 20 Minutes

Servings: 2

Ingredients

1 tablespoon olive oil

1 tablespoon coconut flour

2 cups vegetable broth or water

1cup tempeh

¼ cup Zucchini diced

¼ carrot shredded

¼ cup uncooked wild rice

¼ tablespoon maple syrup

1 teaspoon dried mint

1 teaspoon kosher salt

½ teaspoon pepper

1 clove garlic minced

1 teaspoon cilantro chopped for garnish

Instructions

Add broth, tempeh, zucchini, carrot, wild rice, maple syrup, mint, salt, pepper and minced garlic to the Instant Pot and stir to combine. Secure the lid, making sure the vent is closed.

Using the display panel select the MANUAL or PRESSURE COOK function. Use +/- keys and program the Instant Pot for 15 minutes.

When the time is up, let the pressure naturally release for 10 minutes, then quick-release the remaining pressure.

In a medium bowl, add coconut flour in olive oil until it makes a paste. Ladle 1 cup of the hot soup broth into the paste and stir to incorporate, then pour flour mixture into the Instant Pot.

Using the display panel select CANCEL and then SAUTE. Cook and stir until thickened, then stir in the half and half.

Serve warm topped with chopped cilantro.

Nutrition:

Calories 356, Total Fat 17.8g, Saturated Fat 3.4g, Cholesterol 0mg, Sodium 1957mg, Total Carbohydrate 29.2g ,Dietary Fiber 2.7g, Total Sugars 3.9g ,Protein 24.3g

150. Pear Pumpkin Soup

Preparation Time: 05 Minutes

Cooking Time: 10 Minutes

Servings: 2

Ingredients

½ teaspoon butter

¼ onion finely diced

1 cup pumpkin peeled and cubed

1 pear peeled and cubed

½ teaspoon salt

¼ teaspoon cumin

¼ teaspoon ground coriander

1 cup vegetable broth or water

½ tablespoon coconut cream

½ teaspoon honey

Instructions

Add butter to the Instant Pot. Using the display panel select the SAUTE function.

When butter gets melt, add onions to the Instant pot and sauté until soft, 2-3 minutes. Add pear, salt and spices and stir to combine.

Add broth to the Instant pot then add pumpkin and stir. Turn the Instant pot off by selecting CANCEL, then secure the lid, making sure the vent is closed.

Using the display panel select the MANUAL or PRESSURE COOK function. Use the + /- keys and program the Instant Pot for 5 minutes.

When the time is up, quick-release the remaining pressure, then select CANCEL to turn off the pot.

Use an immersion blender to blend the soup until smooth.

Cool slightly, then stir in coconut cream and honey.

Serve warm.

Nutrition:

Calories 87, Total Fat 2.8g, Saturated Fat 1.6g, Cholesterol 3mg , Sodium 972mg, Total Carbohydrate 13.3g, Dietary Fiber 2.8g , Total Sugars 7.4g, Protein 3.6g

151. Zucchini Coconut Thai Soup

Preparation Time: 15 Minutes

Cooking Time: 20 Minutes

Servings: 2

Ingredients

½ tablespoon Olive oil

½   onion peeled and diced

½ pound Zucchini peeled and diced

1 cup spinach

1 small carrot

1 teaspoon ginger garlic paste

½ tablespoon red curry paste

2 cups vegetable broth or water

½ teaspoon maple syrup

½ cup coconut milk canned

1 tablespoon lime juice

1/4 teaspoon red pepper flakes

1 teaspoon sea salt

1/2 teaspoon black pepper ground

1/4 cup basil

Instructions

Press the Sauté button on the Instant Pot. When display shows 'hot", add olive oil and heat it.

Add the onions and carrots, zucchinis, spinach. Sauté for 3–5 minutes until onions are become translucent.

Add the ginger-garlic paste and curry paste. Continue to sauté for 1 minute.

Add remaining Ingredients, except basil. Close the lid.

Press the Soup button and set time to 20 minutes. When the timer beeps, let pressure release naturally for 10 minutes. Quick release any additional pressure until float valve drops and then unlock lid.

In the Instant Pot, puree soup with a hand blender, or use a stand blender and puree in batches.

Ladle into bowls, garnish each bowl with basil, and serve hot.

Have fun!

Nutrition:

Calories 136, Total Fat 7.2g, Saturated Fat 2.1g, Cholesterol 0mg , Sodium 1930mg, Total Carbohydrate 11.8g, Dietary Fiber 2.3g , Total Sugars 5.7g, Protein 7g

152. Vegetable and Cottage Cheese Soup

Preparation Time: 35 Minutes

Cooking Time: 10 Minutes

Servings: 2

Ingredients

½ (12 ounce) package cottage cheese, drained and cut into ¾-inch cubes

1 tablespoon coconut oil

½ teaspoon dried Italian seasoning

1 diced tomatoes

½ teaspoon basil

1 cup vegetable broth

½ cup fresh peas,

½ cup kale

¼ cup cauliflower

½ cup 1-inch pieces green beans

½ cup chopped green sweet pepper

¼ cup sliced green olives

Shredded Parmesan cheese (optional)

Instructions

Put the cottage cheese in a plastic bag with in a flat plate. Add the oil and Italian season the. Seal bag; Turn to cover the cottage cheese. Marinate in the refrigerator for 2 to 4 hours.

Press the Sauté button on the Instant Pot. When display shows 'hot", add coconut oil and heat it. Press SAUTE function and add cottage chasse and Set timer for 5 min to until cottage cheese browned.

Add Broth and tomato into IP. Then Add peas, kale, cauliflower, green beans and green sweet pepper and again set timer for 10 minutes and close the lid of Instant pot.

When time up .let pressure release naturally for 10 minutes. Quick release any additional pressure until float valve drops and then unlock lid.

Serve the soup and enjoy.

Nutrition:

Calories229, Total Fat 12.3g, Saturated Fat 8.6g, Cholesterol 13mg , Sodium 765mg, Total Carbohydrate 16.9g, Dietary Fiber 4.5g , Total Sugars 6.4g, Protein 15g

153. Zucchini Tomato Soup

Preparation Time: 15 Minutes

Cooking Time: 15 Minutes

Servings: 2

Ingredients

1 pound large tomatoes, cored and cut into pieces

¼   Zucchini, cut into chunks

¼ cup broccoli

1 medium bell pepper, seeded and cut into pieces

1 teaspoon garlic powder

2 tablespoons butter, divided

1 tablespoon vinegar, divided

1 teaspoon plus a pinch of salt, divided

½ teaspoon plus a pinch of ground pepper, divided

¼ avocado

¼ tablespoon chopped fresh basil

Instructions

Cut all the vegetables and set aside.

Press the sauté mode and pour in the butter. When it melt the Add zucchini, broccoli and bell pepper and mix them. Sauté for a few minutes or until the vegetables are tender, about 5 minutes.

Add garlic powder, water and spices and mix.

Close the lid. Set MANUAL COOK or PRESSURE for 4 minutes on HIGH PRESSURE.

Allow the IP to natural release for 5 minutes once timer goes off.

Remove the lid and mix well .Serve soup with topping of avocado and fresh basil.

Have fun!

Nutrition:

Calories 228, Total Fat 17.1g, Saturated Fat 8.4g, Cholesterol 31mg , Sodium 1266mg, Total Carbohydrate 18.5g, Dietary Fiber 6.1g , Total Sugars 10.1g, Protein 4.1g

154. Vegetable Stew

Preparation Time: 15 Minutes

Cooking Time: 15 Minutes

Servings: 2

Ingredients

1 small Onion, minced

1 teaspoon Garlic powder

1 leek, minced

½ Zucchini, minced

1/4 cup Vegetable Broth

2 oz. Button Mushrooms, sliced

1 teaspoon Dried basil

½ teaspoon Italian Seasoning

1/2 teaspoon Salt

1/4 teaspoon Ground Pepper

2 Tomatoes, chopped

1 medium parsnip, chopped

½ yum, chopped

¼ tablespoon Balsamic Vinegar

1 tablespoon Corn-starch

¼ cup green beans

Instructions

Add onion and mushrooms to the Instant Pot inner pot. Press Sauté button and sauté until mushrooms have released their liquid and shrunk in size, about 8 minutes. Stir every couple of minutes.

Add garlic powder and sauté 2 more minutes. Add salt, basil, pepper. Stir. Press Cancel to stop Sauté function. Secure lid in place.

Add all the vegetable in the pot with broth. Press Manual and adjust time to 10 minutes pressure cooking.

Meanwhile add water and corn starch and make a mixer.

When time has lapsed quick release the pressure from the Instant Pot. Remove lid away from you.

Add corn starch mixer into pot and make a thick soup.

Carefully transfer soup into bowl serve and enjoy.

Nutrition:

Calories 158, Total Fat 1.2g, Saturated Fat 0.2g, Cholesterol 1mg , Sodium 714mg, Total Carbohydrate 35.1g, Dietary Fiber 6.4g , Total Sugars 11.1g, Protein 5.5g

155. Jackfruit beetroot Soup

Preparation Time: 10 Minutes

Cooking Time: 20 Minutes

Servings: 2

Ingredients

1 beetroots roughly chopped

½ large green turnips roughly chopped

½ cup jackfruit

2 cup Water cold running tap water

½ teaspoon Ginger powder

2 dried dates

Sea salt to taste

Instructions

Place all the Ingredients into the Instant pot. Pour 2 cups of cold running tap water into the pot. Do not add any salt. Close the lid and pressure cook on manual at High Pressure for 20 minutes. Turn off the heat and fully Natural Release (roughly 20 – 25 minutes).

Carefully open the lid and heat up the pressure cooker to bring the soup back to a full boil. Add sea salt to taste.

Nutrition:

Calories 86, Total Fat 0.3g, Saturated Fat 0.1g, Cholesterol 0mg , Sodium 214mg, Total Carbohydrate 21g, Dietary Fiber 2.6g, Total Sugars 5.5g, Protein 2g

156. Moroccan Veggie Soup

Cooking Time: 45 minutes

Servings: 4

Ingredients

1 2/3 cups chopped tomatoes

1 2/3 chickpeas, drained and rinsed

1 cup loosely spinach, chopped

2 teaspoons vegetable oil

1 onion, chopped

3 celery sticks, chopped

3 garlic cloves, chopped

2 preserved lemons, flesh discarded and rind finely chopped

2 red chili, deseeded and chopped

1 tablespoon tomato purée

2 teaspoons ground cumin

1 teaspoon ground turmeric

½ teaspoon ground cinnamon

1 potato, chopped

1 bunch flat-leaf parsley, chopped

4 tablespoons lemon juice

Instructions

Place a large pan over medium heat. Add onion celery and salt. Cover and cook for 10 minutes.

Add garlic, preserved lemons, red chilies and cook for 2 minutes.

Add tomato puree, spices and cook for 2 minutes.

Add chopped tomatoes, potato, chickpeas and 5 cups of boiling water. Bring to a boil and let it simmer for 30 minutes.

Add spinach, parsley and lemon juice before serving.

157. Tex Mex Black Bean and Avocado Salad

Cooking Time: 15 minutes

Servings: 2

Ingredients

14 oz. black beans, drained and rinsed

3 jars roasted red peppers, chopped

1 avocado, chopped

½ onion, chopped

1 red chili, chopped

1 lime, plus wedges to serve

olive oil

1 teaspoon cumin seeds

2 handfuls rocket

2 pitta breads, warmed

Instructions

Combine beans, peppers, avocado, onion and chili in a large mixing bowl.

Add lime juice, cumin seeds and mix well.

Serve the rocket on two plates with warm pittas and divide the bean mixture.

158. Lentil Fattoush Salad

Cooking Time: 50 minutes

Servings: 2

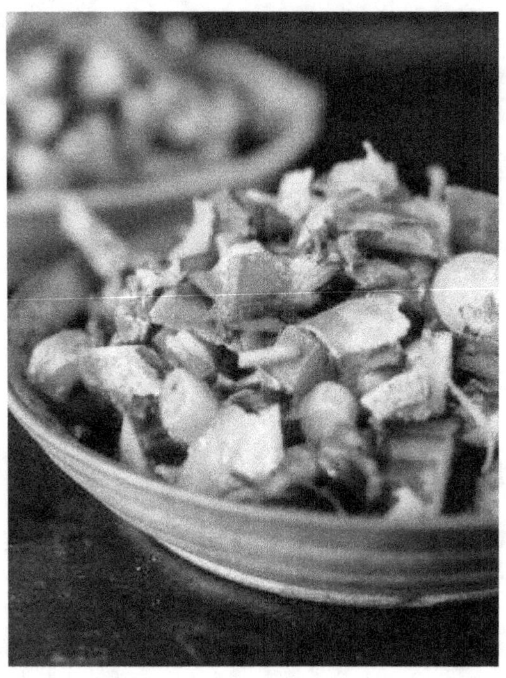

Ingredients

⅓ cup dry green lentils

1 whole wheat pita pocket, chopped into bite sized pieces

2 teaspoons olive oil

2 teaspoons zaatar

4 cups loosely packed arugula

2 stalks celery, chopped

1 carrot stick, chopped

¼ small hothouse cucumber, chopped

1 small radish, thinly sliced

¼ cup dates, chopped

2 tablespoons toasted sunflower seeds

For the maple Dijon vinaigrette:

2 tablespoons olive oil

2 tablespoons balsamic vinegar

1 tablespoon Dijon mustard

1 tablespoon maple syrup

Instructions

Place a small pot over medium heat. Add lentils and 2/3 cup water.

Bring it to a boil, lower the heat and bring it to a simmer for 35 minutes. Remove from the heat and drain excess liquid.

Preheat the oven to 425F. Line a baking sheet with parchment paper.

Mix pita pieces with olive oil and zaatar. Place on a baking sheet and bake for 7 minutes.

Mix arugula, lentils, veggies, dates, sunflower seeds and pita croutons.

Meanwhile in a separate bowl, mix the dressing ingredients and set aside.

Add the dressing and toss well before serving.

159. Sweet Potato Salad

Cooking Time: 35 minutes

Servings: 4

Ingredients

2 sweet potatoes, peeled and cubed

1 tablespoon olive oil

½ teaspoon each of paprika, oregano and cayenne pepper

1 shallot, diced

2 spring onions, chopped

1 small bunch chives, chopped

3 tablespoons red wine vinegar

2 teaspoons olive oil

1 tablespoon pure maple syrup

salt and pepper

Instructions

Preheat the oven to 300F and prepare a baking sheet by lining it with parchment paper.

Place sweet potatoes in the baking sheet.

Drizzle some olive oil and spices, toss well and bake for 30 minutes.

In a separate bowl, mix shallots, scallions, chives, vinegar, olive oil and maple syrup.

Add baked sweet potatoes to the dressing.

160. Lentil Salad with Spinach and Pomegranate

Cooking Time: 15 minutes

Servings: 3

Ingredients

For the vegan lentil salad:

3 cups brown lentils, cooked

1 avocado, cut into slices

2-3 handfuls fresh spinach

½ cup walnuts, chopped

2 apples, chopped

1 pomegranate

For the tahini orange dressing:

3 tablespoons tahini

2 tablespoons olive oil

1 clove of garlic

6 tablespoons water

4 tablespoons orange juice

2 teaspoons orange zest

salt and pepper

Instructions

Prepare lentils according to package instructions.

Place pomegranate in a shallow bowl filled with water, cut in half and take out seeds, remove fibers floating on the water.

Process all dressing ingredients in a food processor. Process until smooth and set aside.

Place salad ingredients in a large bowl and mix well.

Drizzle dressing over salad before serving.

161. Broccoli Salad Curry Dressing

Cooking Time: 30 minutes

Servings: 6

Ingredients

½ cup plain, unsweetened vegan yogurt

¼ cup onion, chopped

2 heads broccoli florets, chopped

2 stalks celery, chopped

½ teaspoon curry powder

¼ teaspoon salt or to taste

2 tablespoons sunflower seeds

Instructions

Mix yoghurt, curry powder and salt.

Toss broccoli florets, celery onion and sunflower seeds.

Drizzle the dressing on top and put the salad in the fridge for 30 minutes.

162. Broccoli Cauliflower Soup

Cooking Time: 35 minutes

Servings: 8

Ingredients

1 medium head broccoli, finely chopped

1 medium head cauliflower, chopped

¼ cup whole wheat pastry flour

4 cups vegetable broth

1 cup unsweetened, unflavored almond milk

1/3 cup nutritional yeast

2 tablespoons olive oil

1 medium onion, chopped

2 cloves garlic, minced

2 carrots, diced

1 potato, diced

1 tablespoon lemon juice

salt and pepper

Instructions

Place a skillet over medium heat. Add oil.

Add and cook onion, salt, pepper for about 5 minutes.

Add garlic and cook for about 1 minute.

Add carrots, broccoli, cauliflower, potato and cook for 5 minutes.

Add flour and mix.

Add broth, almond milk, nutritional yeast and bring the mixture to a boil. Reduce the heat, cover and cook for 20 minutes. Remove from the heat and add lemon juice.

Use immersion blender to blend until chunky before serving.

163. Carrot Ginger Soup

Cooking Time: 50 minutes

Servings: 6

Ingredients

1 lb. carrots, peeled and chopped

3 cups vegetable broth

1 cup vanilla almond milk

1 apple, diced

1 onion, diced

3 tablespoons avocado oil

1 teaspoon garlic, minced

1 tablespoon ginger, minced

½ teaspoon turmeric

Instructions

Preheat the oven to 425F and line a baking sheet with parchment paper.

Place carrots on the baking sheet and drizzle olive oil, salt and pepper. Bake for 30 minutes and set aside to cool.

Combine broth, milk, garlic, ginger, turmeric and vegetables in a food processor. Season with salt and pepper. Pulse until smooth and creamy.

Warm the creamy mixture with carrots on a stove before serving.

164. Persimmon Butternut Squash Soup

Cooking Time: 1 hour

Servings: 4

Ingredients

2 cups butternut squash, peeled and chopped

3 tablespoons olive oil

1 tablespoon butter

½ cup onion, chopped

3 persimmons, peeled and diced

18 oz. vegetable broth

1 cup coconut milk

1/8 teaspoon ground cloves

¼ teaspoon cinnamon

½ teaspoon paprika

¼ teaspoon ground ginger

1 tablespoon maple syrup

salt and pepper

Instructions

Preheat the oven to 400F, Line a baking sheet with parchment paper.

Place squash on the baking sheet and season with oil, cinnamon and salt. Bake for 25 minutes.

Meanwhile place a pot over medium heat.

Add butter and cook onions for 2 minutes.

Add squash, persimmon and cook for 5 minutes.

Add broth, milk, spices, maple syrup and bring it to a boil. Cover, reduce the heat and let it simmer for 20 minutes.

Remove from the heat and blend with an immersion blender until creamy and smooth.

Return to medium heat, add the remaining spices, salt and pepper before serving.

165. Eggplant Tomato Soup

Cooking Time: 35 minutes

Servings: 4

Ingredients

½ cup raw cashews

1 eggplant, cubed

5 large tomatoes, cored and diced

1 onion, chopped

3 garlic cloves

¼ cup extra virgin olive oil

1 ½ cup vegetable broth

1 tablespoon tamari

1 tablespoon fresh oregano

1 tablespoon fresh basil

salt and pepper

Instructions

Preheat the oven to 400F and line a large baking sheet with foil.

Place a small pan over medium heat, add 2 cups water and bring it to a boil. Remove from the heat, add cashews and set aside to soak for 30 minutes.

Place eggplants, tomatoes, onion, garlic and a drizzle of olive oil, salt and pepper. Bake for 20 minutes until tender.

Place baked vegetables, soaked cashews, vegetable broth, tamari herbs and pulse for 1 minute until smooth.

Return to the skillet and heat the soup again before serving.

166. Black Bean Soup

Cooking Time: 35 minutes

Servings: 4

Ingredients

3 15 oz. cans organic black beans

1 15 oz. can organic tomato sauce

¾ cup vegetable broth

1 teaspoon olive oil

1 white onion, chopped

3 cloves garlic, minced

1 ½ tablespoons chili powder

2 teaspoons cumin

1 teaspoon dried oregano

1/8 teaspoon cayenne pepper

salt

Instructions

Place a pot over medium heat, add oil.

Add and cook onions, garlic and cook for 5 minutes.

Add in chili powder, cumin, oregano, cayenne pepper and black pepper.

Add black beans, tomato sauce, broth and cook for 30 seconds. Bring to a boil, reduce the heat and let it simmer for 25 minutes.

167. Mushroom Cream Soup

Preparation Time: 15 Minutes

Cooking Time: 60 minutes

Servings: 6

Ingredients:

2 cups mushrooms, chopped

1 onion, peeled, diced

½ cup coconut cream

1 teaspoon salt

1 teaspoon ground black pepper

1 tablespoon olive oil

2 potatoes, chopped

4 cups of water

Instructions:

Place mushrooms, onion, and olive oil in the instant pot.

sauté the vegetables for 10 minutes or until they are half cooked.

Then add coconut cream, salt, ground black pepper, and potatoes.

Add water and close the lid.

Set sauté mode and cook soup for 50 minutes.

When the time is over and all the ingredients are tender, blend the soup with the help of the hand blender until it is smooth.

Let the cooked soup rest for 10 minutes before serving.

Nutrition:

Calories 128, Carbohydrates 15 g, Fats 7.3 g, Protein 2.6 g

168. Penne Pasta Soup

Preparation Time: 15 Minutes

Cooking Time: 7 minutes

Servings: 2

Ingredients:

1 red bell pepper, chopped

2 cups of water

5 oz penne pasta

1 teaspoon salt

¼ cup fresh dill

1 potato, chopped

1 teaspoon olive oil

½ teaspoon paprika

Instructions:

Cook bell pepper with olive for 3 minutes on sauté mode.

Add penne pasta, potato, paprika, and salt.

Then add water, close and seal the lid.

Cook soup on Manual mode (high pressure) for 7 minutes.

When the time is over, use the quick pressure release.

Chop the dill and add it in the soup. Mix it up and let it rest for 10-15 minutes.

Nutrition:

Calories 325, Carbohydrates 61.8 g, Fats 4.5 g, Protein 11.6 g

169. Winter Stew

Preparation Time: 10 Minutes

Cooking Time: 20 minutes

Servings: 6

Ingredients:

½ cup red lentils

1 cup mushrooms, chopped

1 yellow onion, chopped

2 sweet potatoes, chopped

1 carrot, chopped

½ cup red kidney beans, canned

1 tablespoon tomato paste

2 cups of water

½ cup almond milk

1 teaspoon salt

½ teaspoon peppercorns

1 teaspoon olive oil

Instructions:

Cook mushrooms with onion and olive oil on sauté mode for 10 minutes.

Then add red lentils, sweet potatoes, carrot, red kidney beans, tomato paste, almond milk, water, salt, and peppercorns.

Mix up the ingredients gently.

Close and seal the lid.

Set High-pressure mode and cook the stew for 10 minutes. Then allow natural pressure release.

Mix up the cooked stew carefully.

Nutrition:

Calories 177, Carbohydrates 23.8 g, Fats 5.9 g, Protein 8.8 g

170. Vegan "Beef" Stew

Preparation Time: 10 Minutes

Cooking Time: 45 minutes

Servings: 2

Ingredients:

½ yellow onion, chopped roughly

1 oz celery stalk, chopped

¼ cup carrot, chopped

1 garlic clove, diced

1 tablespoon tomato sauce

¼ cup green peas

1 tomato, chopped

1 cup vegetable stock

1 teaspoon salt

1 teaspoon thyme

2 Yukon potatoes

Instructions:

Chop Yukon potatoes roughly and transfer them in the instant pot.

Add celery stalk, yellow onion, carrot, garlic, tomato sauce, green peas, tomato, salt, thyme, and mix up.

Then add vegetable stock and close the lid.

Set Saute mode and cook the stew for 45 minutes.

When the time is over, check if all the ingredients are cooked and mix up the stew gently.

Nutrition:

Calories 100, Carbohydrates 22.4 g, Fats 1.2 g, Protein 3 g

171. Egyptian Stew

Preparation Time: 10 Minutes

Cooking Time: 12 minutes

Servings: 5

Ingredients:

1 tablespoon tomato paste

1 tablespoon olive oil

1 tablespoon red pepper

1 teaspoon paprika

4 potatoes, peeled, chopped

2 cups lentils

6 cups of water

1 teaspoon salt

1 cup fresh dill, chopped

3 tablespoons lemon juice

Instructions:

Place tomato paste, paprika, potatoes, lentils, water, and salt in the instant pot.

Close and seal the lid.

After this, set Manual mode and cook the stew for 12 minutes.

Then use quick pressure release.

Open the lid and add lemon juice. Mix it up.

Transfer the stew in the serving bowls.

Then mix up together red pepper and olive oil.

Pour the mixture over the stew.

Garnish the meal with fresh dill.

Nutrition:

Calories 451, Carbohydrates 81.1 g, Fats 4.4 g, Protein 25.1 g

172. Moroccan Stew

Preparation Time: 10 Minutes

Cooking Time: 18 minutes

Servings: 4

Ingredients:

1 cup butternut squash, chopped

½ cup chickpeas, canned

1 teaspoon turmeric

1 teaspoon sage

1 teaspoon ground coriander

1 teaspoon thyme

1 teaspoon harissa

1 teaspoon ground ginger

¼ teaspoon saffron

1 lemon slice

1 teaspoon salt

1 teaspoon tomato paste

2 cups of water

Instructions:

In the instant pot, combine together water, tomato paste, salt, saffron, ground ginger, harissa, thyme, ground coriander, sage, turmeric, and canned chickpeas.

Add butternut squash and mix the ingredients.

Add lemon slice and close the lid.

Set Manual mode (high pressure) and cook the stew for 8 minutes. Then allow natural pressure release for 10 minutes more.

Open the lid and chill the stew till the room temperature.

Nutrition:

Calories 117, Carbohydrates 21.1 g, Fats 1.9 g, Protein 5.5 g

173. Peas and Carrot Stew

Preparation Time: 5 Minutes

Cooking Time: 15 minutes

Servings: 5

Ingredients:

3 potatoes, peeled, chopped

2 carrots, chopped

1 cup green peas, frozen

2 cups of water

1 tablespoon tomato paste

1 teaspoon salt

1 teaspoon cayenne pepper

Instructions:

Place carrots, potatoes, and green peas in the instant pot.

Then in the separated bowl combine together tomato paste, water, salt, and cayenne pepper.

Whisk the liquid until it gets a light red color, and then pour it into the instant pot.

Close and seal the lid. Cook the stew on Manual mode for 10 minutes.

Then allow natural pressure release for 5 minutes.

Nutrition:

Calories 125, Carbohydrates 27.5 g, Fats 0.3 g, Protein 4.1 g

174. Mediterranean Vegan Stew

Preparation Time: 10 Minutes

Cooking Time: 35 minutes

Servings: 4

Ingredients:

¼ cup white cabbage, shredded

1 potato, chopped

½ cup corn kernels

1 sweet pepper, chopped

½ cup fresh parsley

1 cup tomatoes, chopped

¼ cup green beans, chopped

1 ½ cup water

1 teaspoon salt

1 tablespoon coconut cream

1 teaspoon white pepper

Instructions:

Place all the ingredients in the instant pot and mix them up.

After this, close the lid and ser sauté mode.

Cook the stew for 35 minutes.

When the time is over, open the lid and mix the stew well.

Check if all the ingredients are cooked and close the lid.

Let the stew rest for 10-15 minutes before serving.

Nutrition:

Calories 83 , Carbohydrates 16.8 g, Fats 1.4 g, Protein 2.8 g

175. Sweet Potato Stew

Preparation Time: 10 Minutes

Cooking Time: 35 minutes

Servings: 2

Ingredients:

¼ cup tomatoes, diced

1 tablespoon wheat flour

1 cup tomato juice

½ onion, diced

1 tablespoon olive oil

1 tablespoon chives, chopped

1 teaspoon salt

1 teaspoon curry powder

3 sweet potatoes, roughly chopped

½ cup of water

1 teaspoon sugar

Instructions:

Pour olive oil in the instant pot. Add diced onion and sweet potatoes.

Sprinkle the vegetables with salt, curry powder, and cook on sauté mode for 10 minutes.

After this, whisk together wheat flour and water until smooth.

Pour the liquid in the instant pot.

Add tomato juice and sugar.

Close the lid and cook the stew on sauté mode for 35 minutes. Mix up the stew every 10 minutes.

Check if the sweet potatoes are cooked and add chopped chives. Mix up the stew well.

Nutrition:

Calories 165, Carbohydrates 24.7 g, Fats 7.4 g, Protein 2.6 g

176. Kuru Fasulye

Preparation Time: 15 Minutes

Cooking Time: 20 minutes

Servings: 4

Ingredients:

1 cup cannellini beans

6 cups of water

2 tablespoons tomato paste

1 onion, diced

1 bell pepper, chopped

1 teaspoon coconut oil

1 teaspoon chili flakes

1 teaspoon ground black pepper

1 teaspoon salt

1 teaspoon cayenne red pepper

Instructions:

Cook diced onion and bell pepper with coconut oil on sauté mode for 3 minutes.

Add tomato paste and cannellini beans.

Mix up the ingredients and add water, chili flakes, ground black pepper, and red pepper.

Close and seal the lid.

Set Manual mode (high pressure) and cook the meal for 15 minutes.

Then allow natural pressure release for 15 minutes more.

Nutrition:

Calories 193, Carbohydrates 34.5 g, Fats 1.8 g, Protein 11.9 g

177. Rainbow Stew

Preparation Time: 10 Minutes

Cooking Time: 30 minutes

Servings: 4

Ingredients:

1 eggplant, sliced

1 zucchini, sliced

2 tomatoes, sliced

½ cup corn kernels

¼ cup red beans, canned

1 cup of water

1 tablespoon coconut oil

1 teaspoon salt

1 teaspoon paprika

1 teaspoon cayenne pepper

Instructions:

In the mixing bowl combine together sliced eggplant, zucchini, corn kernels, salt, paprika, and cayenne pepper. Shake the mixture well.

After this, transfer the vegetables in the instant pot.

Add coconut oil, water, and red beans.

Close the lead and cook the stew on sauté mode for 30 minutes.

Then open the lid, stir the meal gently and let it rest with the opened lid for 5 minutes.

Nutrition:

Calories 135, Carbohydrates 22 g, Fats 4.3 g, Protein 5.6 g

178. Irish Stew

Preparation Time: 20 Minutes

Cooking Time: 50 minutes

Servings: 4

Ingredients:

1 cup baby potatoes

1 cup mushrooms, roughly chopped

1 oz parsnip, chopped

2 cups of water

1 tablespoon tomato paste

1 tablespoon coconut cream

1 teaspoon dried dill

1 teaspoon dried coriander

1 teaspoon salt

1 tablespoon tomato sauce

1 teaspoon olive oil

¼ cup baby carrot, chopped

1 cup beer

Instructions:

Cook baby potatoes with olive oil on sauté mode until potatoes are light brown.

Then add mushrooms, parsnip, tomato paste, coconut cream, dried dill, coriander, salt, and tomato sauce.

Add baby carrots and mix up the stew well.

Then add beer and water. Close the lid.

Set Saute mode and cook the stew for 50 minutes.

When the time is over, switch off the instant pot and let stew rest for 15 minutes.

Nutrition:

Calories 85 , Carbohydrates 11.2 g, Fats 2.2 g, Protein 1.8 g

179. Fennel Soup

Preparation Time: 10 Minutes

Cooking Time: 8 minutes

Servings: 2

Ingredients:

1 cup of coconut milk

½ cup almond milk

8 oz fennel bulb, chopped

1 cup cauliflower, chopped

1 garlic clove, diced

1 tablespoon fresh dill, chopped

½ teaspoon chili pepper

1 teaspoon salt

Instructions:

Pour coconut milk and almond milk in the instant pot.

Add chopped fennel bulb, cauliflower, garlic clove, chili pepper, and salt.

Close and seal the lid.

Cook the soup on High-pressure mode for 8 minutes.

Then use quick pressure release.

Open the lid and blend the soup until smooth.

Ladle it into the soup bowls and sprinkle with fresh dill.

Nutrition:

Calories 360, Carbohydrates 23.1 g, Fats 3.2 g, Protein 6.1 g

180. African Stew

Preparation Time: 20 Minutes

Cooking Time: 60 minutes

Servings: 4

Ingredients:

¼ cup peanuts, chopped

3 tablespoons peanut butter

1 teaspoon garlic, diced

1 teaspoon minced ginger root

1 cup collard greens, chopped

3 yams, chopped

1 white onion, roughly chopped

1 teaspoon cumin

1 teaspoon ground black pepper

1 teaspoon onion powder

1 teaspoon cayenne pepper

1 teaspoon oregano

1 teaspoon cilantro

1 bell pepper, chopped

2 cups of water

½ cup almond milk

1 tablespoon almond butter

Instructions:

sauté yams, onion, minced ginger root, and diced garlic with almond butter for 5 minutes. Stir the mixture from time to time.

Meanwhile, mix up together all the spices; cilantro, oregano, cayenne pepper, onion powder, ground black pepper, and cumin.

Add the spice mixture in the instant pot.

Then add bell pepper, peanuts, and peanut butter.

Add almond milk and water.

Check if you add all the ingredients and close the lid.

Set saute mode and cook stew for 50 minutes.

When the time is over, switch off the instant pot and let the stew stay for at least 15 minutes more.

Nutrition:

Calories 288, Carbohydrates 22.9 g, Fats 20.5 g, Protein 8.6 g

181. Thai Curry Soup

Preparation Time: 10 Minutes

Cooking Time: 13 minutes

Servings: 4

Ingredients:

6 oz firm tofu, cubed

1 teaspoon curry paste

1 teaspoon curry powder

½ cup of coconut milk

2 cups of water

1 tablespoon fish sauce

2 tablespoons soy sauce

1 teaspoon paprika

2 cups mushroom, chopped

1 teaspoon almond butter

2 tablespoons lemon juice

¼ teaspoon grated lime zest

Instructions:

On the sauté mode, cook mushrooms with curry powder, curry paste, fish sauce, soy sauce, paprika, and almond butter for 10 minutes. Mix up the mushrooms well.

Ten add cubes tofu, coconut milk, and grated lime zest.

Close and seal the lid.

Cook the soup on high-pressure mode for 3 minutes. Then make quick pressure release and open the lid.

Add lemon juice and mix up soup gently.

Nutrition:

Calories 150, Carbohydrates 6.2 g, Fats 12.2 g, Protein 7.1 g

182. Garden Stew

Preparation Time: 10 Minutes

Cooking Time: 24 minutes

Servings: 3

Ingredients:

1 cup green beans, chopped

1 potato, chopped

4 oz asparagus, chopped

1 large tomato, chopped

1 cup vegetable broth

1 teaspoon ground black pepper

1 teaspoon almond butter

½ cup kale, chopped

¼ cup spinach, chopped

Instructions:

Place all the ingredients except spinach and kale in the instant pot and close the lid.

Cook the ingredients on Manual mode for 4 minutes. Then allow natural pressure release for 5 minutes.

Open the lid and add spinach and kale. Mix up the stew well.

Close the lid and keep cooking stew on sauté mode for 10 minutes more.

When the time is over, switch off the instant pot and let stew rest for 10 minutes before serving.

Nutrition:

Calories 127, Carbohydrates 19.4 g, Fats 3.8 g, Protein 6.4 g

183. Tom Yum Soup

Preparation Time: 15 Minutes

Cooking Time: 16 minutes

Servings: 4

Ingredients:

3 cups of water

2 tablespoons Tom Yum paste

1 teaspoon lemongrass

¼ teaspoon ground ginger

1 teaspoon garlic, diced

2 tomatoes, chopped

4 oz green beans, chopped

2 oz celery stalk, chopped

1 carrot, chopped

1 cup spinach, chopped

¼ cup bok choy, chopped

Instructions:

In the instant pot combine together water, Tom Yam paste, lemongrass, ground ginger, garlic, and chopped tomatoes.

Close and seal the lid. Cook mixture on Manual mode for 4 minutes.

Then make a quick pressure release and open the lid.

Add green beans, celery stalk, carrot, and bok choy.

Mix the soup up and add spinach.

Close the lid and cook soup on sauté mode for 16 minutes.

Then let the cooked soup rest for 10 minutes with the closed lid.

Nutrition:

Calories 62, Carbohydrates 8.6 g, Fats 2.5 g, Protein 1.6 g

184. Coconut Cream Soup

Preparation Time: 15 Minutes

Cooking Time: 7 minutes

Servings: 5

Ingredients:

5 cups of coconut milk

1 cup of water

2 cups carrots

1 onion, diced

1 teaspoon salt

1 teaspoon turmeric

1 teaspoon white pepper

Instructions:

Peel and chop carrots.

Cook the diced onion with salt, turmeric, and white pepper in the instant pot for 2 minutes.

Then stir the vegetable carefully and add water, coconut milk, and chopped carrot.

Close and seal the lid.

Set High-pressure mode and cook soup for 7 minutes. After this, allow natural pressure release for 10 minutes.

Open the lid and blend the soup with immersion blender until smooth.

Nutrition:

Calories 581, Carbohydrates 20.2 g, Fats 57.3 g, Protein 6.2 g

185. Hot Pepper Chickpea Stew

Preparation Time: 15 Minutes

Cooking Time: 15 minutes

Servings: 3

Ingredients:

1 cayenne pepper, chopped

1 cup chickpea

4 cups of water

1 tablespoon almond butter

1 onion, chopped

2 cups spinach, chopped

1 tablespoon coconut yogurt

1 teaspoon salt

Instructions:

Place almond butter in the instant pot and melt it on saute mode.

Add spinach and chopped cayenne pepper.

Then add onions and chickpeas.

Sprinkle the ingredients with salt and add water.

Close and seal the lid.

Cook stew on Manual mode for 15 minutes.

Then allow natural pressure release for 15 minutes.

Transfer the cooked stew in the serving bowls, add coconut yogurt and mix it up.

Nutrition:

Calories 297, Carbohydrates 45.9 g, Fats 7.2 g, Protein 15.1 g

186. Summer Stew

Preparation Time: 15 Minutes

Cooking Time: 7 minutes

Servings: 6

Ingredients:

1 eggplant, chopped roughly

1 cup bok choy, chopped

1 cup spinach, chopped

½ cup fresh cilantro, chopped

1 red onion, cut into petals

2 sweet peppers, chopped

½ cup of rice

5 cups vegetable broth

1 teaspoon salt

1 teaspoon thyme

1 teaspoon dried parsley

Instructions:

Put eggplant, bok choy, spinach, cilantro, onion, and sweet peppers in the instant pot.

Add rice, vegetable broth, salt, thyme, and dried parsley.

Mix up the vegetables with the help of the spoon. Close and seal the lid.

Set Manual mode (high pressure) and cook the stew for 7 minutes.

When the time is over, allow natural pressure release for 10 minutes.

Mix up the stew before serving.

Nutrition:

Calories 131, Carbohydrates 22.9 g, Fats 1.6 g, Protein 6.9 g

187. Texas Stew

Preparation Time: 10 Minutes

Cooking Time: 5 minutes

Servings: 2

Ingredients:

¼ cup green chili, canned, chopped

½ cup tomatoes, canned, diced

½ teaspoon salt

1/3 cup corn kernels, frozen

½ cup potatoes, chopped

½ cup kidney beans, canned

½ cup almond milk

1 teaspoon dried parsley

Instructions:

Combine together all the ingredients in the instant pot.

Close and seal the lid.

Cook stew on Manual mode for 5 minutes. After this, allow natural pressure release for 5 minutes.

Chill the stew till the room temperature.

Transfer the stew in the serving bowls.

Nutrition:

Calories 359, Carbohydrates 46 g, Fats 15.2 g, Protein 13.6 g

188. Soybean Stew

Preparation Time: 20 Minutes

Cooking Time: 20 minutes

Servings: 4

Ingredients:

1 cup soybeans, soaked

¼ cup tomatoes, chopped

3 cups of water

1 teaspoon mustard

1 zucchini, chopped

1 tablespoon soy sauce

1 jalapeno pepper, sliced

3 oz vegan Parmesan, grated

Instructions:

Place soybeans and tomatoes in the instant pot.

Add mustard, zucchini, soy sauce, jalapeno pepper, and close the lid.

Set Manual mode (High pressure) and cook the stew for 20 minutes.

Then allow natural pressure release for 20 minutes.

Transfer the cooked stew in the serving bowls and top with grated cheese.

Nutrition:

Calories 289, Carbohydrates 21.2 g, Fats 9.6 g, Protein 26.8 g

189. Iranian Stew

Preparation Time: 15 Minutes

Cooking Time: 6 minutes

Servings: 4

Ingredients:

1 cup parsley, chopped

½ cup fresh cilantro, chopped

½ cup spinach, chopped

½ cup kale, chopped

½ lime

1 eggplant, chopped

1 yellow onion, chopped

1 cup red kidney beans, canned

2 cups vegetable broth

1 teaspoon harissa

2 teaspoons paprika

1 tablespoon almond butter

Instructions:

Put parsley, cilantro, spinach, kale, and chopped onion in the instant pot.

Add red kidney beans, vegetable broth, paprika, harissa, and almond butter.

Add eggplant.

Close and seal the lid.

Cook the stew for 6 minutes in Manual mode. After this, allow natural pressure release for 10 minutes.

Open the lid and mix up the stew carefully.

It is recommended to serve stew warm.

Nutrition:

Calories 259, Carbohydrates 42.7 g, Fats 4.2 g, Protein 16.2 g

190. Coated Halloumi Sticks

Preparation Time: 5 minutes

Cooking time: 10 minutes

Servings: 6

Ingredients:

1/3 cup almond flour

2 tsp smoked paprika

1 lb halloumi cheese, cut into 2-inch strips

½ cup grated Monterey Jack cheese

2 tbsp chopped parsley

½ tsp cayenne powder

Directions:

Preheat the oven to 350 F and grease a baking sheet with cooking spray.

In a small bowl, mix the almond flour with paprika. Lightly coat the halloumi in the mixture and arrange on the baking sheet.

In a smaller bowl, mix the remaining Ingredients and sprinkle over the halloumi cheese.

Bake the cheese in the oven for 10 minutes or until golden brown.

Remove allow cooling for 3 minutes and serve warm.

Nutrition:

Calories:396, Total Fat:29.3g, Saturated Fat:18.3g, Total Carbs:11g, Dietary Fiber:1g, Sugar:9g, Protein:23g, Sodium:1944mg

191. Fried Avocados

Preparation Time: 5 minutes

Cooking time: 2 minutes

Servings: 6

Ingredients:

½ cup olive oil

3 large avocados, halved and pitted

1 ½ tbsp almond flour

Salt and black pepper to taste

1 cup grated Pecorino Romano cheese

2 large eggs

Directions:

Heat the olive oil in a deep-frying pan over medium heat.

Meanwhile, slice the avocados into 6 pieces each and set aside.

In a bowl, mix the almond flour, salt, black pepper, and cheese. Set aside.

Crack the eggs into a medium bowl and lightly whisk

Coat the avocado slices in the egg and then generously cover with the cheese mixture.

Fry in the hot oil until golden brown, 1 to 2 minutes, and transfer to a wire rack.

Cool for 1 minute and serve immediately.

Nutrition:

Calories:523, Total Fat:51.7g, Saturated Fat:7.7g, Total Carbs:14g, Dietary Fiber:10g, Sugar:2g, Protein:6g, Sodium:47mg

192. Spicy Mozzarella Bites

Preparation Time: 5minutes

Cooking time: 5minutes

Servings: 4

Ingredients:

1 cup olive oil, for frying

1 cup almond flour

½ tsp chili powder

1 tsp onion powder

1 tsp garlic powder

1 tsp dried basil

1 large egg

1 cup almond meal

1 cup mozzarella cheese cubes

Directions:

Heat the olive oil in a deep-frying pan.

Meanwhile, in a medium bowl, mix the almond flour, chili powder, onion powder, garlic powder, and basil. Set aside.

Lightly beat the egg in a small bowl and pour the almond meal in a plate.

Coat each mozzarella cube in the almond flour mixture, then in the eggs, and then lightly in the almond meal.

Fry in the hot oil until golden brown on both sides, then transfer to a wire rack to drain grease.

Serve the cheese bites warm.

Nutrition:

Calories540:, Total Fat:55.5g, Saturated Fat:7.9g, Total Carbs:3g, Dietary Fiber:1g, Sugar:g1, Protein:10g, Sodium:224mg

193. Seeds Flapjacks

Preparation Time: 5 minutes

Cooking time: 25 minutes

Servings: 4

Ingredients:

6 tbsp unsalted butter

8 tbsp sugar-free maple syrup

8 tbsp erythritol

3 tbsp sesame seeds

3 tbsp chia seeds

3 tbsp flax seeds

1 tbsp poppy seeds

3 tbsp hemp seeds

3 tbsp sunflower seeds

4 tbsp dried goji berries, chopped

Directions:

Preheat the oven to 350 F and line a baking sheet with baking paper.

Melt the butter, maple syrup, and erythritol in a small saucepan over low heat while gently stirring and occasionally until the erythritol dissolves.

Take the pan off the heat and stir in the remaining Ingredients.

Spread the mix onto the baking sheet and bake in the oven for 20 minutes or until golden brown.

Remove after and slice the flapjacks into 16 strips. Cool slightly and turn the flapjacks onto a chopping board. Divide into squares and cool completely.

Serve.

Nutrition:

Calories:283, Total Fat:26.4g, Saturated Fat:8.7g, Total Carbs:9g, Dietary Fiber:3g, Sugar:4g, Protein:7g, Sodium:13mg

194. Zucchini Chips with Seeds

Preparation Time: 5 minutes

Cooking time: 10 minutes

Servings: 4

Ingredients:

4 large zucchinis, thinly sliced

4 tbsp olive oil

1 tsp smoked paprika

2 tbsp hemp seeds

2 tbsp poppy seeds

1 tsp red chili flakes

Directions:

Preheat the oven to 350 F and place the zucchini in a colander. Sprinkle with salt and allow liquid draining for 5 minutes. Pat the zucchinis dry with a paper towel and transfer to a baking sheet.

Drizzle with olive oil, sprinkle with the paprika, and massage to spice on top.

Scatter with the seeds and chili flakes on top and season with salt, black pepper, and roast in the oven for 20 minutes or until golden brown and crispy.

Transfer to a serving bowl and serve warm.

Nutrition:

Calories173:, Total Fat:17.7g, Saturated Fat:2.3g, Total Carbs:3g, Dietary Fiber:2g, Sugar:0g, Protein:2g, Sodium:8mg

195. Herby Cheesy Nuts

Preparation Time: 5 minutes

Cooking time: 15 minutes

Servings: 4

Ingredients:

1 egg white

4 tsp yeast extract

1 tsp erythritol

2 cups mixed nuts

Sea salt and black pepper to season

3 tbsp grated Pecorino Roman cheese

½ tsp dried parsley

Directions:

Preheat the oven to 350 F.

In a large bowl, beat the egg white, yeast extract, and erythritol.

Mix in the nuts and spread on a baking sheet. Bake in the oven for 10 minutes.

In a small bowl, mix the salt, black pepper, cheese, and parsley.

Remove the nuts after and toss in the cheese mixture. Bake further for 5 minutes or until sticky and brown.

Transfer to a serving bowl; allow cooling for 5 minutes, and enjoy.

Nutrition:

Calories517:, Total Fat:51.9g, Saturated Fat:8.7g, Total Carbs:12g, Dietary Fiber:6g, Sugar:4g, Protein:9g, Sodium:263mg

196. Chocolate Pecan Biscuits

Preparation Time: 10minutes| Cooking time: 20minutes

Servings: 4

Ingredients:

4 oz butter, softened

2 tbsp erythritol

2 tbsp sugar-free maple syrup

1 egg

1 tsp vanilla extract

½ cup almond flour

½ tsp baking soda

2/3 cup unsweetened chocolate chips

½ cup chopped walnuts

Directions:

Preheat the oven to 350 F and lightly grease a baking sheet with cooking spray.

In a medium bowl, whisk the butter, erythritol, and maple syrup until smooth. Beat in the egg and mix in the vanilla extract.

In another bowl, mix the almond flour with baking soda and mix into the wet Ingredients. Fold in the chocolate chips and pecans.

Add tablespoons of the batter onto the baking sheet, creating 2-inch spaces in between each spoon, and press each dough to slightly flatten.

Bake in the oven for 10 to 15 minutes or until cooked.

Allow cooling in the oven for 5 minutes then transfer to a wire rack to cool completely.

Serve.

Nutrition:

Calories288:, Total Fat:30.6g, Saturated Fat:15.5g, Total Carbs:2g, Dietary Fiber:1g, Sugar:0g, Protein:3g, Sodium:355mg

197. Broccoli Chips with Cheese Dip

Preparation Time: 15minutes

Cooking time: 20minutes

Servings 6

Ingredients:

For the broccoli chips:

1 medium head broccoli, cut into florets

1 ½ cup water, for steaming

½ tsp salt or to taste

1 ½ tbsp flaxseed meal

1 tbsp flax seeds

1 tbsp chia seeds

For the cheese dip:

8 oz cream cheese, softened

2 tbsp sugar-free maple syrup

¼ cup toasted almonds, finely chopped

¼ cup toasted pecans, finely chopped

3 tbsp chia seeds

1 tbsp lemon zest

Directions:

For the broccoli chips:

Preheat the oven to 350 F.

Pour the broccoli and water into a medium pot and bring to boil over medium heat the broccoli softens. Drain through a colander and transfer to a food processor; puree until very smooth.

Pour the mixture into a medium bowl and stir in the salt and flaxseed meal until evenly combined. Mix in the flax seeds and chia seeds too.

Line a large baking sheet with baking paper and spread the batter on the sheet. Cover with a plastic wrap and use a rolling pin to flatten and level the mixture evenly and lightly.

Take off the plastic wrap after and use a knife to cut our chip-size squares on the batter.

Bake in the oven for 15 to 20 minutes or until the chips are golden brown and crispy.

Remove from the oven, allow cooling for 5 minutes and transfer to a serving bowl.

For the cheese dip:

In a medium bowl, mix the cream cheese and maple syrup until properly combined.

Fold in the remaining Ingredients and spoon the dip into serving bowls.

Serve the dip with the chips.

Nutrition:

Calories:435, Total Fat:32.8g, Saturated Fat:11.9g, Total Carbs:27g, Dietary Fiber:16g, Sugar:5g, Protein:15g, Sodium:596mg

198. Pesto Mushroom Pinwheels

Preparation Time: 15 minutes

Cooking time: 25 minutes

Servings: 4

Ingredients:

For the puff pastry:

¼ cup almond flour + extra for dusting

3 tbsp coconut flour

½ tsp xanthan gum

½ tsp salt

4 tbsp cashew cream, room temperature

1/4 teaspoon baking soda

¼ cup of butter, cold

3 whole eggs

3 tbsp erythritol

1 ½ tsp vanilla extract

1 whole egg, beaten

For the filling:

1 cup basil pesto (olive oil base)

2 cups baby spinach, steamed

2/3 cup canned mixed mushrooms, drained and chopped

Salt and black pepper to taste

1 cup grated cheddar cheese

1 egg, beaten for brushing

Directions:

In a large bowl, mix the almond flour, coconut flour, xanthan gum, and salt.

Add the cashew cream, baking soda, and butter; mix with an electric hand mixer until crumbly. Add the erythritol and vanilla extract until mixed in. Then, pour in 3 of the eggs one after another while mixing until formed into a ball.

Flatten the dough a clean flat surface, cover in plastic wrap, and refrigerate for 1 hour.

After, lightly dust a clean flat surface with almond flour, unwrap the dough, and roll out into 15 X 12 inches. Spread the pesto on top with a spatula leaving a 2-inch border on one end.

In a bowl, combine the spinach and mushrooms, season with salt and black pepper, and spread the mixture on the pesto. Sprinkle with the cheddar cheese and roll up as tightly as possible from a shorter end. Chill in the refrigerator for 10 minutes.

Meanwhile, preheat the oven to 380 F.

Remove the pastry onto a flat surface and use a sharp knife to into 24 slim discs. Arrange on the baking sheet, brush with the remaining egg, and bake in the oven for 20 to 25 minutes or until golden.

Transfer onto a plate, allow cooling for 5 minutes, and serve with tomato dipping sauce.

Nutrition:

Calories:741, Total Fat:76.1g, Saturated Fat:18.9g, Total Carbs:11g, Dietary Fiber:3g, Sugar:3g, Protein:14g, Sodium:210mg

199. Berry Trail Mix Bars

Preparation Time: 10 minutes

Cooking time: 15 minutes

Servings: 4

Ingredients:

2 cups mixed nuts

¼ cup coconut chips

1 egg, beaten

½ cup butter, melted

¼ cup mixed seeds

Salt to taste

1 cup mixed dried berries

Directions:

Preheat the oven to 350 F and line a baking sheet with parchment paper.

In a food processor, pulse the nuts for 1 to 2 minutes until roughly chopped.

Transfer to a large bowl and stir in the coconut chips, egg, butter, salt, mixed seeds, and dried berries.

Spread the mixture in the baking sheet into an even layer and bake for 15 to 20 minutes or until golden brown.

Cool afterward and cut into bars.

Nutrition:

Calories:406, Total Fat:41.2g, Saturated Fat:9g, Total Carbs:9g, Dietary Fiber1:g, Sugar:2g, Protein:4g, Sodium:359mg

200. Spicy Cashew Dip

Preparation Time: 5 minutes

Servings: 4

Ingredients:

3 oz. toasted cashews + a little for garnishing

3 tbsp coconut cream

¼ cup water

½ lemon, juiced

½ tsp smoked paprika

Cayenne pepper to taste

½ tsp salt

½ cup olive oil

Directions:

Process all the Ingredients in a high-speed blender until smooth.

Dish the dip and enjoy!

Nutrition:

Calories:755, Total Fat:82.2g, Saturated Fat:9.5g, Total Carbs:7g, Dietary Fiber:2g, Sugar:4g, Protein:1g, Sodium:421mg

201. Yellow Squash Nacho Chips

Preparation Time: 6minutes

Cooking Time: 20minutes

Servings

Ingredients:

1 large yellow squash

Salt to season

1 ½ cups avocado oil

1 tbsp taco seasoning

Directions:

With a mandolin slicer, cut the squash into thin, round slices and place in a colander.

Sprinkle the squash with a lot of salt and allow sitting for 5 minutes to drain liquid. After, press the water out of the squash and pat dry with a paper towel.

Pour the avocado oil into a deep skillet and heat over medium heat.

In batches, fry the squash pieces in the oil until golden brown and crispy, 10 minutes.

Use a slotted spoon to remove the squash onto a paper towel-lined plate.

Sprinkle the chips with taco seasoning and serve.

Nutrition:

Calories:591, Total Fat:57g, Saturated Fat:19.6g, Total Carbs:20g, Dietary Fiber:12g, Sugar:2g, Protein:9g, Sodium:219mg

202. Guacamole Hummus

Preparation Time: 12 minutes

Cooking Time 15 minutes | Serving: 4

Ingredients:

3 large avocados, pitted and peeled

½ cup freshly chopped parsley + extra for garnishing

½ cup butter

1 garlic clove, minced

½ tsp coriander powder

¼ cup pumpkin seeds

¼ cup sesame paste

Juice from ½ lemon

Salt and black pepper to taste

Directions:

Add all the Ingredients to a food processor and blend until smooth.

Spoon the guacamole hummus and serve.

Nutrition:

Calories:520, Total Fat:46.4g, Saturated Fat:10.7g, Total Carbs:16g, Dietary Fiber:5g, Sugar:1g, Protein:18g, Sodium:687mg

203. Mixed Seed Crackers

Preparation Time: 12 minutes

Cooking Time: 45 minutes

Servings: 6

Ingredients:

1/3 cup sesame seed flour

1 ½ cups mixed seeds

1 tbsp psyllium husk powder

1 tsp salt

¼ cup butter, melted

1 cup boiling water

Directions:

Preheat the oven to 300 F.

In a medium bowl, combine the sesame seed flour, seeds, psyllium husk powder, and salt.

Pour in the butter and hot water and mix until dough forms with a gel-like consistency.

Line a baking sheet with parchment paper and place the dough on the sheet. Cover the dough with another parchment paper and with a rolling pin flatten the dough into the baking sheet. Remove the parchment paper on top.

Bake in the oven for 45 minutes while paying close attention to prevent the seeds from burning.

Turn the oven off and allow the crackers to cool and dry in the oven, 10 minutes.

Remove the sheet and break the crackers into small pieces. Serve.

Nutrition:

Calories:310, Total Fat:31.1g, Saturated Fat:7.3g, Total Carbs:5g, Dietary Fiber:1g, Sugar:1g, Protein:5g, Sodium:758mg

204. Kale Dip

Preparation Time: 15 minutes

Cooking Time: 20 minutes

Servings: 4

Ingredients:

2 oz. frozen chopped kale

2 tbsp olive oil

2 tbsp dried cilantro

1 tbsp dried oregano

1 tsp garlic powder

½ tsp salt

¼ tsp black pepper

1 cup vegan mayonnaise

4 tbsp coconut cream

Juice of ½ a lemon

Directions:

Add all the Ingredients to a food processor and blend until smooth.

Allow the dip to sit for about 10 minutes for the flavors to develop.

Pour the dip into a serving bowl and enjoy!

Nutrition:

Calories:369, Total Fat:31.5g, Saturated Fat:18.6g, Total Carbs:10g, Dietary Fiber:1g, Sugar:2g, Protein:13g, Sodium:804mg

205. Tofu Stuffed Peppers

Preparation Time: 5 minutes

Cooking Time: 20 minutes

Servings: 4

Ingredients:

1 cup mini red and yellow bell peppers

1 oz. tofu, chopped into small bits

1 tbsp chopped fresh parsley

1 cup cream cheese

½ - 1 tbsp chili paste, mild

2 tbsp melted butter

Cooking spray

1 cup shredded Parmesan cheese

Directions:

Preheat the oven to 400 F.

Use a knife to cut the bell peppers into two (lengthwise) and remove the core.

In a bowl, mix the tofu with the parsley, cream cheese, chili paste, and melted butter until smooth.

Fill the bell peppers with the mixture and use the back of the spoon to level the filling in the peppers.

Grease a baking sheet with cooking spray and arrange the stuffed peppers on the sheet.

Sprinkle the Parmesan cheese on top and bake the peppers for 15 to 20 minutes until golden brown and the cheese melted.

Remove onto a serving platter and serve warm.

Nutrition:

Calories:611 , Total Fat:51.1g, Saturated Fat:21.4g, Total Carbs: 9g, Dietary Fiber:2g, Sugar: g, Protein: g30, Sodium:1084 mg

206. Loaded Vegan Bacon Bake

Preparation Time: 5 minutes

Cooking Time: 46 minutes

Servings: 4

Ingredients:

1 large cauliflower head, cut into florets

6 slices vegan bacon, chopped

2 tbsp olive oil

1 lb tofu

2 tbsp butter

1 cup coconut cream

2 oz cream cheese, softened

1 ¼ cups grated cheddar cheese

Salt and black pepper to taste

¼ cup chopped scallions

Directions:

Preheat the oven to 300 F.

Fill a large pot with water, two-thirds way up and bring to a boil over medium heat. Pour the cauliflower into the pot and blanch for 2 minutes. Drain through a colander and set aside.

Place the vegan bacon into a medium pot and fry on both sides until browned and crispy, 7 minutes. Spoon into a plate and set aside.

Heat the olive oil in the pot, add and cook the tofu until browned, 10 minutes. Spoon onto a plate and set aside.

Add the butter, coconut cream, cream cheese, two-thirds of the cheddar cheese, salt, and black pepper to the pot and melt the Ingredients over medium heat while often stirring, 7 minutes.

Arrange the cauliflower florets in a baking dish, pour the cream mixture over, and scatter the top with the vegan bacon and scallions.

Sprinkle the remaining cheddar cheese on top, and bake in the oven until the cheese is bubbly and golden, 30 minutes.

Remove the dish, spoon the dish into serving plates, and serve immediately.

Nutrition:

Calories:308 , Total Fat:24.1g, Saturated Fat:11.5g, Total Carbs: 6g, Dietary Fiber:1g, Sugar: 3g, Protein: 20g, Sodium: 447mg

207. BBQ Seitan Burgers

Preparation Time: 10 minutes

Cooking Time: 10 minutes |Serving Size: 4

Ingredients:

1 lb crumbled seitan

1 tsp salt

1 tsp black pepper

1 tsp onion powder

2 tsp garlic powder

1 tbsp smoked paprika

2 tbsp unsweetened tomato paste

¼ cup white vinegar

2 tbsp tamari sauce

½ cup vegetable broth

¼ cup melted butter

¼ cup baby spinach

4 low carb hamburger buns, halved

4 slices cheddar cheese

Directions:

In a medium bowl, mix all the Ingredients up to the butter and mold 4 to 6 patties from the mixture.

Melt the butter in a medium skillet and fry the patties on both sides until golden brown, 10 minutes.

Divide the spinach in the bottom layer of each low carb bun, place a patty on each and top with a cheddar cheese slice each. Cover the buns and serve immediately.

Nutrition:

Calories:352 , Total Fat:27.6g, Saturated Fat:7.9g, Total Carbs: 19g, Dietary Fiber:6g, Sugar: 12g, Protein: 9g, Sodium: 263mg

208. Tofu Portobello Cheeseburgers

Preparation Time: 15 minutes

Cooking Time: 15 minutes |Serving Size: 6

Ingredients:

1 lb tofu block, pressed and crumbled

Salt and black pepper to taste

1 tbsp sugar-free Worcestershire sauce

1 tbsp coconut oil

6 large Portobello caps, destemmed, rinsed, and patted dry

6 slices Gouda cheese

For topping:

6 lettuce leaves

6 large tomato slices

¼ cup mayonnaise

Directions:

In a medium bowl, combine the tofu, salt, black pepper, and Worcestershire sauce. Using your hands, mold 6 patties out of the mixture, and set aside.

Heat the coconut oil in a medium skillet; place in the Portobello caps and cook until softened, 3 to 4 minutes. Remove onto serving plates and set aside.

Put the tofu patties in the skillet and cook on both sides until brown and compacted, 10 minutes. Place the Gouda cheese slices on the tofu, allow melting for 1 minute and lift each tofu patty onto each mushroom cap.

Divide the lettuce on top, the tomato slices, and top with some mayonnaise.

Serve immediately.

Nutrition:

Calories:396 , Total Fat: 29.3g, Saturated Fat:18.3 g, Total Carbs: 11g, Dietary Fiber:1 g, Sugar: 9g, Protein: 23g, Sodium: 1944 mg

209. Enchilada Style Vegan Bacon Stuffed Pepper

Preparation Time: 15 minutes

Cooking Time: 53 minutes

Servings: 6

Ingredients:

6 large bell peppers, mixed colors

1 ½ tbsp olive oil

Salt and black pepper to taste

3 tbsp butter, room temperature

½ white onion, chopped

3 cloves garlic, minced

4 slices vegan bacon (chopped into small cubes)

3 tsp enchilada seasoning

1 cup cauliflower rice

¼ cup grated cheddar cheese

Sour cream for serving

Directions:

Preheat the oven to 400 F and grease a baking dish with cooking spray. Set aside.

Cut the peppers at the head and scoop out the seeds and membrane to make cups. Drizzle with the olive oil and some salt. Set aside.

Melt the butter in a large skillet; add and sauté the onion and garlic for 3 minutes. Stir in the vegan bacon, enchilada seasoning, salt, and black pepper. Cook until the vegan bacon browns, 10 minutes.

Mix in the cauliflower rice until adequately incorporated. Turn the heat off.

Spoon the mixture firmly into the peppers, divide the cheddar cheese on top, and put the stuffed peppers in the baking dish. Bake in the oven for 40 minutes or until the cheese is bubbly and melted.

Remove the peppers, plate, and top with some sour cream.

Serve warm.

Nutrition:

Calories:520 , Total Fat:46.4g, Saturated Fat:10.7g, Total Carbs: 16g, Dietary Fiber:5g, Sugar: 1g, Protein: 18g, Sodium: 687mg

210. Popcorn

Preparation Time: 05 Minutes

Cooking Time: 15 Minutes

Servings: 2)

Ingredients

1-1/2 tablespoons avocado oil

½ cup popcorn kernels

1 teaspoon salt

Instructions

Select SAUTE button and adjust until light is on MORE. Wait till the display indicates HOT.

Add avocado oil and leave it to melt completely. Add salt. Start by adding a few popcorn kernels inside the pot and wait until it pops (cover glass lid on top). This might take a few seconds. Popcorn kernels will heat up and then pop.

When you see couple of them pop, add rest of popcorn kernels. Place the glass lid on top leaving slightly ajar for steam to escape.

Lift the inner pot and shake briefly once after 30 seconds or so.

Popcorn will start popping after 3 to 4 minutes. The popping will continue.

Once the popping slows down, when you can count 3 between pops, remove the inner pot from the cooker and let it sit for 1 or 2 minutes. Un-popped kernels will pop. You want to have 'almost' all popcorn kernels to pop.

Swirl the pop once again. Transfer to serving popcorn tubs and serve immediately.

Nutrition:

Calories 113, Total Fat 1.9g, Saturated Fat 0.1g, Cholesterol 0mg, Sodium 775mg, Total Carbohydrate 26g , Dietary Fiber 5.5g , Total Sugars 0g, Protein 3.6g

211. Crispy Tofu

Preparation Time: 05 Minutes

Cooking Time: 15 Minutes

Servings: 2)

Ingredients

1cup tofu, cut into pieces for your choice

Salt and freshly-cracked black pepper

1 tablespoon butter

½ cup tomato sauce

½ tablespoon lime juice

Chopped fresh cilantro

Instructions

In a medium mixing bowl, whisk together the tomato sauce , lime juice combined. Set aside until ready to use.

Season tofu pieces on all sides with salt and pepper.

Click the "Sauté" setting on the Instant Pot. Add the butter, followed tofu — turning every 45-60 seconds or so — until the tofu is browned on all sides. Transfer tofu to a separate clean plate, and repeat with the remaining tofu, searing until it has browned on all sides. Press "Cancel" to turn off the heat.

Pour in the tomato sauce mixer, and toss briefly to combine with the tofu. Close lid securely and set vent to "Sealing"

Cook on high pressure for 2 minutes, followed by a natural release (about 15 minutes).

Sprinkle with chopped fresh cilantro, then serve and enjoy.

Nutrition:

Calories159, Total Fat 11.2g, Saturated Fat 4.8g, Cholesterol 15mg , Sodium 382mg, Total Carbohydrate 6.7g, Dietary Fiber 2.4g , Total Sugars 3.6g, Protein 11.4g

212. Broccoli Little Flower

Preparation Time: 10 Minutes

Cooking Time: 12 hr

Servings: 2

Ingredients

1 medium head broccoli

2 tablespoons tomato sauce

1 tablespoon butter

1 tablespoon lemon juice

1 tablespoon red chilli

1 teaspoon cumin

½ teaspoon cinnamon

Instructions

Chop the broccoli into florets that are about the size of the tip of your thumb.

In a large bowl, combine broccoli and remaining Ingredients. Toss to coat evenly.

Divide the broccoli onto the cooking trays in an even layer.

Place the drip pan in the bottom of the cooking chamber and insert one cooking tray in the top-most position and one tray in the bottom-most position.

Using the display panel, select DEHYDRATE, then adjust the temperature to 130 degrees and the time to 12 hours, then touch START.

When the Dehydrate program is complete, remove it and serve immediately.

Nutrition:

Calories 78, Total Fat 6.2g, Saturated Fat 3.7g, Cholesterol 15mg , Sodium 139mg, Total Carbohydrate 5.1g, Dietary Fiber 1.9g, Total Sugars 1.6g, Protein 1.9g

213. Baked Sweet potato

Preparation Time: 05 Minutes

Cooking Time: 20 Minutes

Servings: 2)

Ingredients

1 cup water

2 sweet potato

1 teaspoon butter

Pinch salt

Pinch Paprika

Instructions

Place 1 cup water in the bottom of the Instant pot.

Place a rack or steamer basket over the water .Wash and pat dry the sweet potatoes. Poke with a fork in 3-4 places each.

Rub each with a little butter and salt, paprika generously.

Place the sweet potatoes in the steamer basket and set pressure cook setting to high.

Pressure cook on high for 16 minutes.

Let pressure release naturally for the best results.

To crisp the skin (optional) place them directly on the rack in a hot convection or toaster oven for a few minutes.

Nutrition:

Calories 120, Total Fat 2.1g, Saturated Fat 1.2g, Cholesterol 5mg, Sodium 136mg, Total Carbohydrate 23.6g, Dietary Fiber 3.8g, Total Sugars 7.4g, Protein 2.3g

214. Orange Tofu Lettuce Wraps

Preparation Time: 05 Minutes

Cooking Time: 20 Minutes

Servings: 2

Ingredients

1 cup tofu, cut into 2-inch cubes

1 tablespoon corn-starch

1 tablespoon coconut oil

1/3 cup water

¼ tablespoon soy sauce

½ teaspoon honey

¼ teaspoon Chile-garlic sauce

2 tablespoons fresh orange juice

1 teaspoon grated orange zest

Salt and freshly ground black pepper

1 or 2 small heads leafy green, or romaine lettuce leaves, for serving

Thinly sliced cucumbers carrots, red bell pepper, carrot,

Fresh herbs like Thai basil cilantro, mint

Instructions

Toss the tofu with ½ tablespoon corn-starch in a bowl to coat evenly. Select Sauté on the Instant Pot and warm the coconut oil. Cook the tofu, turning as every minute or so the tofu doesn't stick to the pan, until all sides are golden brown, about 5-6 minutes

Add the water, soy sauce, honey, Chile-garlic sauce, and 1 tablespoon of the orange juice and stir to mix well.

Lock the lid in place and turn the valve to Sealing Press the keep Warm/Cancel button to reset the program, then press the pressure button and set the cook time for 7 minutes at high pressure.

Let the steam release naturally for about 10 minutes, then turn the valve to Venting to release any residual steam. Carefully remove the lid and transfer about ¼ cup of the sauce to a small bowl.

Add the remaining reaming corn-starch to the bowl and stir to dissolve. Return the mixture to theInstant pot and stir well. Press the Keep Warm/Cancel button to reset the program, then press the Sauté button and cook, stirring occasionally, until the sauce thickens, about 5 minutes. Stir in the remaining 1tablespoon orange juice and the orange zest and season with salt and pepper.

Arrange the lettuce leaves on a large serving platter with the sliced garnishes and herbs, and serve.

Nutrition:

Calories 194, Total Fat 12.3g, Saturated Fat 7g , Cholesterol 0mg, Sodium 133mg, Total Carbohydrate 13.5g, Dietary Fiber 2.1g, Total Sugars 6.1g, Protein 11.6g

215. Oregano Tofu balls

Preparation Time: 15 Minutes

Cooking Time:15 Minutes

Servings: 2

Ingredients

1 egg

1tablespoon coconut milk

¼ cup quick-cooking oats

2 tablespoons thinly sliced green onions

½ small red bell pepper finely chopped

¼ teaspoon salt

¼ teaspoon black pepper

½ teaspoon oregano

¼ cup finely shredded sharp cheddar cheese

1 cup tofu crumbled

1 tablespoon avocado oil

1 ½ cups water

Instructions

In a large bowl lightly beat egg and coconut milk together. Add oats, green onions, bell peppers, salt, pepper, oregano and cheese, stir to thoroughly mix. Add crumbled tofu, mix well.

Using a spoon shape tofu mixture into balls. Turn on the Sauté function on Instant Pot. Once pot is hot, add 1 avocado oil. Sauté the tofu balls, carefully turning occasionally so they brown on all sides (approx. 8-10 mins). Once browned remove meatballs from the Instant Pot and set aside.

Add 1 ½ cups of water to the Instant Pot. Place a steamer basket (or trivet) in the Instant Pot. Arrange browned tofu balls on the rack, stacking as necessary to fit all tofu balls in the pot.

Set Instant Pot to MANUAL/PRESSURE COOK on High Pressure for 2 minutes. Once cooking cycle is complete do a QUICK RELEASE to remove pressure from the pot. Serve immediately. Sprinkle with additional oregano if desired.

Nutrition:

Calories 251, Total Fat 15.5g, Saturated Fat 6.6g, Cholesterol 97mg , Sodium 450mg, Total Carbohydrate 12.3g, Dietary Fiber 3.4g, Total Sugars 2.5g, Protein 18.6g

216. Garlic Chili Potatoes

Preparation Time: 05 Minutes

Cooking Time: 15 Minutes

Servings: 2

Ingredients

½ tablespoon avocado Oil

1 Dry Red Chili whole

½ teaspoon Garlic powder

½ cup onions sliced

½ bell pepper choice of colour

1 tablespoon chili paste

¼ teaspoon Soy sauce

Salt adjust to taste

1 cup baby Potatoes

1 green onions chopped, divided

¼ tablespoon Corn-starch

1/3 cup Water

1 teaspoon Honey optional

1 teaspoon Sesame seeds to garnish

Instructions

Add baby potatoes and water in Instant pot Select High pressure and Set timer for 10 minutes. Once cooking cycle is complete do a QUICK RELEASE to remove pressure from the pot. Set aside

Select Sauté mode in Instant pot and heat avocado oil .Add dried red chili, garlic powder and onions. Sauté for 2-3 minutes until the onions become transparent and start to lightly brown.

Add bell peppers and sauté for another minute. Add soy sauce, honey, red chili paste, salt and stir well. Add the boiled potatoes and sauté for 4-5 mins. Stir frequently and scrape off from the bottom of the pot.

Mix the corn starch in the water until it forms a smooth texture. Add it in to the potatoes along with half of the green onions. Lock the lid and set

MANUAL/PRESSURE COOK on High Pressure for 2 minutes. Once cooking cycle is complete do a QUICK RELEASE to remove pressure from the pot.

Garnish with sesame seeds and green onions. Serve immediately.

Nutrition:

Calories 82, Total Fat 2.6g , Saturated Fat 0.2g , Cholesterol 3mg , Sodium 133mg, Total Carbohydrate 13.9g, Dietary Fiber 1.9g , Total Sugars 7.7g, Protein 2g

217. Candied Almonds

Preparation Time: 05 Minutes

Cooking Time: 15 Minutes

Servings: 2

Ingredients

¼ cup water

¼ cup honey

¼ tablespoon ground nutmeg

½ cup whole almonds

Instructions

Combine the water, honey, and nutmeg ,almonds in Instant Pot. Cover the Instant Pot and lock it in. Make sure the vent on top is set to "sealing". Set manual or pressure cook timer for 2 minutes.

Once timer reaches zero, quick release the pressure.

Pour the almonds onto a baking sheet lined with waxed paper. Separate almonds using forks. Allow to cool about 15 minutes.

Nutrition:

Calories 271, Total Fat 12.2g, Saturated Fat 1.1g, Cholesterol 0mg , Sodium 3mg, Total Carbohydrate 40.4g, Dietary Fiber 3.2g, Total Sugars 36.1g, Protein 5.2g

218. Black beans with Fresh Dill and Parsley

Preparation Time: 10 Minutes

Cooking Time: 25 Minutes

Servings: 2

Ingredients

½ cup black beans Dried

1 tablespoons coconut oil

1 tablespoon fresh parsley Stems removed chopped

1 tablespoon fresh dill Stems removed chopped

1 leek Chopped

½ carrot Peeled and sliced

½ cup sweet corn

1 bay leaves

2 Slices of Orange With peel and flesh

½ tablespoon tomato paste

¼ teaspoon salt

¼ teaspoon pepper

1-1/2 cups Water

Instructions

Wash the black beans very well and pick out any stones.

Add all of the Ingredients to the Instant Pot and stir well.

Cover the Instant Pot and lock it in.

Make sure the vent on top is set to "sealing". Set manual or pressure cook timer for 25 minutes.

Once timer reaches zero, quick release the pressure.

Enjoy!

Nutrition:

Calories 147, Total Fat 7.4g, Saturated Fat 6g, Cholesterol 0mg , Sodium 329mg, Total Carbohydrate 22g, Dietary Fiber 6.3g , Total Sugars 4.5g, Protein 4.5g

219. Loaded Mashed Broccoli

Preparation Time: 10 Minutes

Cooking Time: 15 Minutes

Servings: 2

Ingredients

1 medium head broccoli cut into florets

1 cup water

½ tablespoon coconut oil

½ tablespoon coconut cream

Salt

½ teaspoon garlic minced

1/4 teaspoon mustard powder

1/4 teaspoon chili powder

1/4 teaspoon pepper

1/8 cup shredded goat cheese

1/4 cup grated mozzarella

2 leek parts only, sliced

Instructions

Pour 1 cup of water in the pot, followed by steam rack.

Load broccoli florets into a steamer basket and lower on to steam rack, then secure the lid, making sure the vent is closed.

Using the display panel select the MANUAL or PRESSURE COOK function. Use the +/- keys and program the Instant Pot for 3 minutes.

Meanwhile, add Mash Mixture Ingredients to a food processor or blender.

When cooking time is up, quick-release the pressure.

Carefully drain the cooking liquid and transfer broccoli to the food processor or blender. Process to desired consistency and adjust seasonings as needed.

Transfer the broccoli to a 7' x 11" baking dish or shallow casserole.

Top with goat cheeses and mozzarella . Set under a broiler 5-7 minutes or until cheese is lightly browned.

Remove from oven and allow to cool slightly until set. Sprinkle leek over the top and serve.

Nutrition:

Calories76, Total Fat 5.9g, Saturated Fat 4.6g, Cholesterol 4mg, Sodium 128mg, Total Carbohydrate 4.1g, Dietary Fiber 1.5g , Total Sugars 1g, Protein 3.1g

220. **Cabbage with Balsamic Vinegar**

Preparation Time: 10 Minutes

Cooking Time: 15 Minutes

Servings: 2

Ingredients

1 cabbage halved lengthwise

½ cup water

1 tablespoon coconut oil

½ garlic powder

½ tablespoon balsamic vinegar

¼ teaspoon salt

¼ teaspoon freshly ground black pepper

1 tablespoon roasted Poppy seeds.

Instructions

Place the cabbage in the steamer basket. Pour the water into the inner pot, and place the trivet inside. Place the basket on the trivet. Lock the lid into place. Select Steam, and set the time to 1 minute. Make sure the steam release knob is in the sealed position.

After cooking, Quick Release the pressure. Unlock and remove the lid. Using tongs, carefully transfer the cabbage to a serving plate. Discard the water, and wipe the inner pot dry.

Select Sauté, and pour in the coconut oil. Once hot, add the garlic powder and sauté for 1 minute. Add the cabbage, vinegar, salt, and pepper, and sauté for 2 minutes. Sprinkle with the roasted poppy seed and serve hot.

Nutrition:

Calories 99, Total Fat 9.1g, Saturated Fat 6.2g, Cholesterol 0mg , Sodium 301mg, Total Carbohydrate 4.4g, Dietary Fiber 1.8g , Total Sugars 1.6g, Protein 1.5g

221. Cilantro Lime tofu

Preparation Time: 0 Minutes

Cooking Time: 20 Minutes

Servings: 2

Ingredients

1 tablespoon coconut oil

1 cup tofu

½ teaspoon garlic powder

¼ cup vegetable broth

1 tablespoon lime juice

¼ teaspoon red chilli

¼ teaspoon salt

1 tablespoon chopped cilantro

Additional chopped cilantro for garnish

Instructions

Add coconut oil to the Instant Pot. Using the display panel select the SAUTE function.

When oil gets hot, brown the tofu on 2 sides, 1 minutes per side.

Add garlic powder and cook for 1-2 minutes more.

Add vegetable broth and lime juice to the pot and deglaze by using a wooden spoon to scrape the brown bits from the bottom of the pot.

Sprinkle red chilli, salt and cilantro over the top. Do not stir. Turn the pot off by selecting CANCEL, then secure the lid, making sure the vent is closed.

Using the display panel select the MANUAL or PRESSURE COOK function. Use the + /- keys and program the Instant Pot for 5 minutes.

When the time is up, let the pressure naturally release for 15 minutes, then quick-release the remaining pressure.

Serve warm sprinkled with additional cilantro.

Nutrition:

Calories 162, Total Fat 12.2g, Saturated Fat 7g , Cholesterol 0mg , Sodium 402mg, Total Carbohydrate 5g, Dietary Fiber 1.4g, Total Sugars 1.4g, Protein 11.3g

222. Ranch Cauliflower

Preparation Time: 05 Minutes

Cooking Time: 20 Minutes

Servings: 2

Ingredients

1 head cauliflower, cut into 1" pieces

½ teaspoon dried basil

Salt

1 teaspoon garlic minced

¼ cup vegetable broth

½ cup mozzarella cheese shredded

½ tablespoon ranch dressing

Instructions

Add cauliflower, basil, salt, minced garlic and vegetable broth to the pot. Deglaze by using a wooden spoon to scrape the brown bits from the bottom of the pot. Then secure the lid, making sure the vent is closed.

Using the display panel select the MANUAL or PRESSURE COOK function. Use the + /- keys and program the Instant Pot for 5 minutes.

When the time is up, quick-release the remaining pressure.

Add the cheese, ranch dressing. Stir to combine.

Serve hot.

Nutrition:

Calories 41, Total Fat 0.3g, Saturated Fat 0.1g, Cholesterol 0mg , Sodium 234mg, Total Carbohydrate 7.8g, Dietary Fiber 3.4g , Total Sugars 3.4g, Protein 3.4g

223. Honey BBQ Jackfruit

Preparation Time: 05 Minutes

Cooking Time: 25Minutes

Servings: 2

Ingredients

1 cup Jackfruit

½ cup BBQ sauce

¼ cup water

¼ cup brown sugar

1/8 cup maple syrup

1 tablespoon Worcestershire sauce

½ tablespoon garlic powder

¼ teaspoon paprika

Instructions

Add BBQ Sauce, water, brown sugar, maple syrup to the Instant Pot and stir to combine. Add the jackfruit pieces and stir to coat.

Secure the lid, making sure the vent is closed.

Using the display panel select the MANUAL function. Use the + /- keys and program the Instant Pot for 10 minutes.

When the time is up, quick-release the remaining pressure.

Remove the jackfruit pieces to a foil-lined baking sheet and brush with additional BBQ sauce.

Set pan under the broiler until sauce is bubbly, 2 minutes.

Nutrition:

Calories307, Total Fat 0.5g, Saturated Fat 0.1g, Cholesterol 0mg , Sodium 793mg, Total Carbohydrate 76.6g, Dietary Fiber 2g , Total Sugars 47.6g, Protein 1.6g

224. Mini Tempeh Quiche

Preparation Time: 10 Minutes

Cooking Time: 10 Minutes

Servings: 2

Ingredients

¼ cup feta cheese shredded

½ cup tempeh finely diced

1 teaspoon chives snipped

1 tablespoon kale leaves cut into thin ribbons

1 egg beaten

¼ tablespoon coconut cream

½ teaspoon garlic powder

¼ teaspoon salt

1 cup Water

Additional feta cheese for garnish

Instructions

Coat the inside of a silicone mold with non-stick spray

Firmly press the feta cheese into the bottom and slightly up the sides of the silicone mold. Top with diced tempeh, chives and kale.

Combine the egg, coconut cream, garlic powder and salt in a medium bowl and whisk thoroughly. Pour into molds. Molds should not be more than 3/4 full.

Pour 1 cup of water in the Instant Pot and insert the trivet. Carefully lower the mold on to the trivet. Secure the lid, making sure the vent is closed.

Using the display panel select the MANUAL or PRESSURE COOK function*. Use the +/- buttons and program the Instant Pot for 5 minutes.

When the time is up, let the pressure naturally release for 5 minutes, then quick-release the remaining pressure.

Carefully remove the mold and turn out onto a plate while still warm. Immediately flip each mini quiche so that the mushrooms are on top and press down lightly with fingers to flatten the bottom of each quiche.

Garnish with additional feta cheese if desired. Serve warm.

Nutrition:

Calories 232, Total Fat 16.2g, Saturated Fat 8.4g, Cholesterol 120mg, Sodium 805mg, Total Carbohydrate 6.7g, Dietary Fiber 0.2g , Total Sugars 2.2g, Protein 16.7g

225. Kale Artichoke Dip

Preparation Time: 02 Minutes

Cooking Time: 05 Minutes

Servings: 2

Ingredients

½ cup artichoke hearts drained 1 can or 1 jar

½ small onion finely diced

1/8 cup vegetable broth

½ teaspoon garlic powder

1 cup kale

1 tablespoon Cheddar cheese

¼ tablespoon coconut cream

¼ cup Greek yogurt

½ cup shredded parmesan

½ cup shredded mozzarella

1 teaspoon hot sauce or to taste

Instructions

Mix together drained artichoke hearts, onion, vegetable broth and garlic powder in the Instant Pot.

Top with frozen kale, cheddar cheese, coconut cream and Greek yogurt. Do not stir.

Secure the lid, making sure the vent is closed.

Using the display panel select the MANUAL or PRESSURE COOK function. Use the + /- keys and program the Instant Pot for 4 minutes.

When the time is up, quick-release the remaining pressure.

Stir in cheese and (optional hot sauce). Serve with tortilla chips

Nutrition:

Calories 96, Total Fat 3.4g, Saturated Fat 2.2g, Cholesterol 9mg , Sodium 313mg, Total Carbohydrate 10.1Dietary Fiber 1.5g, Total Sugars 3.7g, Protein 6.5g

226. Crispy Edamame

Preparation Time: 02 Minutes

Cooking Time: 15 Minutes

Servings: 2

Ingredients

½ cup shelled edamame

¼ tablespoon butter

1/4 tablespoon grated feta cheese

Salt and pepper to taste

Instructions

Add butter, edamame, salt, pepper and feta cheese to the Instant Pot and stir to combine. Secure the lid, making sure the vent is closed.

Using the display panel select the MANUAL function. Use the + /- keys and program the Instant Pot for 05 minutes.

When the time is up, quick-release the remaining pressure.

Nutrition:

Calories 61, Total Fat 3.6g , Saturated Fat 1.3g , Cholesterol 5mg , Sodium 27mg, Total Carbohydrate 3.4g, Dietary Fiber 1.1g , Total Sugars 0.8g, Protein 4g

227. Caramelized Pumpkin Seeds

Preparation Time: 10 Minutes

Cooking Time: 15 Minutes

Servings: 2

Ingredients

1 tablespoon honey

1/8 teaspoon cumin

¼ teaspoon ground nutmeg

¼ teaspoon ginger powder

1 pinch cayenne pepper

1cup raw whole pumpkin seeds, washed and dried

¼ teaspoons salt, or to taste

½ tablespoon coconut oil

Instructions

In a large bowl, stir together honey, cumin seed, ground nutmeg, ginger powder, and cayenne pepper, and set aside.

Add coconut oil in instant pot when hot . Add pumpkin seeds and sprinkle with salt to taste. Add honey mixture in the instant pot. Lock the lid.

Press Pressure cook on Max pressure for 5 minutes with the Keep Warm setting off.

Serve

Nutrition:

Calories 64, Total Fat 3.6g, Saturated Fat 3g, Cholesterol 0mg, Sodium 1mg, Total Carbohydrate 9.1g, Dietary Fiber 0.2g , Total Sugars 8.7g, Protein 0.1g

228. Classic Texas Caviar

Preparation Time: 10 Minutes

Cooking Time: 15 Minutes

Servings: 2

Ingredients

½ cup black-eyed peas,

¼ cup diced tomatoes,

½ small onion, cut into small dice

½ yellow bell pepper, stemmed, seeded and cut into small dice

¼ tablespoon chopped fresh cilantro

1 tablespoon red wine vinegar

1 tablespoon coconut oil

¼ teaspoon salt

¼ teaspoon ground black pepper

1/4 teaspoon garlic minced

½ teaspoon dried oregano

½ teaspoon ground cumin

Instructions

Pour the water into the instant pot and then place the black-eyed peas.

Lock the lid into place, making sure the nozzle is in the sealing position.

Use the Manual setting and set the timer for 15 minutes. Use the natural release method when the timer is up.

When all the pressure is out of your instant pot, carefully remove the lid

Mix all Ingredients in a medium bowl; cover and refrigerate 2 hours or up to 2 days. Before serving, adjust seasonings to taste, adding extra vinegar, salt and pepper. Transfer to a serving bowl.

Nutrition:

Calories 130, Total Fat 7.6g, Saturated Fat 5.9g, Cholesterol 0mg , Sodium 307mg, Total Carbohydrate 13.6g, Dietary Fiber 3.4g, Total Sugars 2.9g, Protein 3.8g

229. Zucchini Chips

Preparation Time: 10 Minutes

Cooking Time: 15 Minutes

Servings: 2

Ingredients

1 medium zucchini, cut into 1/4-inch slices

¼ cup seasoned dry bread crumbs

1/8 teaspoon ground black pepper

2 tablespoons grated feta cheese

1 egg white

2 tablespoon coconut oil

Instructions

In one small bowl, stir together the bread crumbs, pepper and feta cheese. Place the egg white in a separate bowl. Dip zucchini slices into the egg whites, then coat the breadcrumb mixture.

Select Sauté and adjust to High heat Instant pot. Add coconut oil when it hot add zucchini chips until browned and crispy.

Nutrition:

Calories 224, Total Fat 16.6g, Saturated Fat 13.4g, Cholesterol 9mg, Sodium 395mg, Total Carbohydrate 14.1g, Dietary Fiber 1.9g, Total Sugars 3.1g, Protein 6.5g

230. 21Glazed Teriyaki Potato

Preparation Time: 00 Minutes

Cooking Time: 30 Minutes

Servings: 2

Ingredients

Sauce

1 tablespoon soy sauce

¼ tablespoon honey

½ teaspoon rice vinegar

½ teaspoon garlic powder

½ teaspoon ginger powder

½ teaspoon toasted sesame oil

½ teaspoon pepper

½ teaspoon Sriracha sauce or to taste

1 cinnamon stick

potato

1 cup baby potatoes

1 teaspoon corn starch

1 tablespoon Water

Sesame seeds and sliced green onions for garnish

Instructions

Combine Sauce Mixture Ingredients in the Instant Pot and stir to combine.

Add baby potato and toss to coat, then secure the lid, making sure the vent is closed.

Using the display panel select the MANUAL or PRESSURE COOK function. Use the + /- keys and program the Instant Pot for 5 minutes.

When the time is up, let the pressure naturally release for 15 minutes, then quick-release the remaining pressure.

Carefully remove the potato from the pot to a foil-lined baking sheet coated with non-stick spray and set aside.

Turn the Instant pot off by selecting CANCEL, then using the display panel select the SAUTE function.

In a small bowl, mix together ¼ cup cooking liquid with corn-starch. Stir into the pot.

Continue to cook and stir until sauce is thickened and reduced, 3-5 minutes.

Add the potatoes with the sauce and set under the broiler until caramelized, 7-12 minutes.

Serve potatoes garnished with sesame seeds and sliced green onions, with remaining sauce for dipping on the side.

Nutrition:

Calories 48, Total Fat 1.2g, Saturated Fat 0.2g, Cholesterol 0mg, Sodium 458mg, Total Carbohydrate 8.7g, Dietary Fiber 1.4g 5%, Total Sugars 2.5g, Protein 1.3g

231. Broccoli with Blue Cheese

Preparation Time: 05 Minutes

Cooking Time:02 Minutes

Servings: 2

Ingredients

1 cup water

1 cup broccoli

1 teaspoon coconut oil

½ tablespoon balsamic vinegar

1 tablespoon crumbled blue cheese

1 tablespoon crushed Peanuts

Instructions

Add water to the Instant Pot. Place broccoli evenly in steamer basket and place basket in pot. Lock lid.

Press the Manual or Pressure Cook button and adjust cook time to 2 minute. Quick release pressure until float valve drops and then unlock lid.

Transfer broccoli to a serving dish and toss with oil and vinegar. Garnish with blue cheese and peanuts. Serve warm.

Nutrition:

Calories 51, Total Fat 3.6g, Saturated Fat 2.8g, Cholesterol 3mg , Sodium 78mg, Total Carbohydrate 3.2g, Dietary Fiber 1.2g, Total Sugars 0.8g, Protein 2.2g

232. Lemon Ginger Cauliflower

Preparation Time: 05 Minutes

Cooking Time:02 Minutes

Servings: 2

Ingredients

1 medium head cauliflower

1 cup water

1 tablespoon butter

2 teaspoons freshly squeezed lemon juice

½ teaspoon salt

1 teaspoon ginger powder

Instructions

Place the cauliflower in a steamer basket and put the basket into the Instant Pot. Add the water. Lock the lid and turn the steam release handle to Sealing. Using the Manual or Pressure Cook function, set the cooker to Low Pressure for 02 minutes.

When the cook time is complete, quick release the pressure.

In a serving bowl, stir together the oil, lemon juice, salt, and ginger powder.

Carefully remove the lid and add the cauliflower to the bowl. Toss to combine. Taste and add the remaining lemon juice and/or ginger, as needed.

Nutrition:

Calories 127, Total Fat 6.1g, Saturated Fat 3.8g, Cholesterol 15mg, Sodium 713mg, Total Carbohydrate 16g , Dietary Fiber 7.3g , Total Sugars 7g, Protein 5.9g

233. Nutmeg Orange Pumpkin

Preparation Time: 10 Minutes

Cooking Time:05 Minutes

Servings: 2

Ingredients

1 cup pumpkin peeled and cut in 1-inch cubes

¼ cup orange juice

¼ tablespoon orange zest

½ tablespoon maple syrup

½ teaspoon salt

½ teaspoon nutmeg

1 tablespoon coconut oil

Instructions

Place pumpkin in Instant Pot; stir in the orange juice, orange zest, maple syrup, salt, and nutmeg. Place lid on Instant pot and lock into place to seal. Pressure Cook or Manual on High Pressure for 5 minutes. Use Quick Pressure Release. Press Cancel.

Carefully drain liquid from the pot. Turn pot to High Sauté, add the coconut oil and stir into pumpkin until melted. Press Cancel.

Nutrition:

Calories 104, Total Fat 7.1g, Saturated Fat 6.1g, Cholesterol 0mg , Sodium 583mg, Total Carbohydrate 10.8g, Dietary Fiber 0.5g , Total Sugars 6.5g, Protein 0.8g

234. Cabbage Hash

Preparation Time: 05 Minutes

Cooking Time: 10 Minutes

Servings: 2

Ingredients

1 small red onion peeled and sliced

1 small sweet potato peeled and small-diced

½ cabbage trimmed and halved

1 cup water

1 tablespoon honey

1 tablespoon fresh pomegranate juice

1/8 teaspoon hot sauce

½ tablespoon chopped fresh basil

Instructions

Press the Sauté button on the Instant Pot. Add onion, sweet potato, and cabbage to the Instant Pot and stir-fry Add water to Instant pot and insert steamer basket. Add veggies to basket. Lock lid.

Press the Manual or Pressure Cook button and adjust cook time to 3 minutes. When timer beeps, quick-release pressure until float valve drops and then unlock lid.

Transfer cooked veggies to a serving dish. Toss with honey, pomegranate juice, and hot sauce. Garnish with basil. Serve warm.

Nutrition:

Calories71, Total Fat 0g, Saturated Fat 0g, Cholesterol 0mg , Sodium 18mg, Total Carbohydrate 18g, Dietary Fiber 1.6g 6%, Total Sugars 12.8g, Protein 0.8g

235. Smoky Nuts and Brussel Sprouts

Preparation Time: 4 minutes

Cooking Time: 4 minutes

Servings: 4

Ingredients:

½ tsp liquid smoke

¼ cup water

2 cups baby Brussels sprouts

1 tbsp vegan butter

¼ cup mixed almonds and pecans

2 tbsp maple syrup

Salt to taste

Instructions:

Open the instant pot and pour in the liquid smoke and water. Stir.

Fit a steamer basket over the water and pour in the Brussel sprouts.

Close the lid, secure the pressure valve, and select Steam mode. Cook for two minutes.

Once the timer is done, perform a quick pressure release, and open the lid.

Remove the steamer basket with greens and pour out the water.

Select Sauté mode on the pot and add the vegan butter to melt. Return the Brussels sprouts to the pot, add the almond, pecans and maple syrup. Cook further until the nuts are tender and season with salt.

Turn the pot off and spoon the snack into serving bowls. Enjoy.

Nutrition:

Calories 88, Carbohydrates 11.5 g, Fats 4.6 g, Protein 2.6 g

236. Tofu Balls in Cranberry Sauce

Preparation Time: 10 minutes

Cooking Time: 10 minutes

Servings: 4

Ingredients:

1 (14 oz) firm tofu

1 medium white onion, diced

1 garlic clove, crushed

1 tbsp dried oregano

Salt and black pepper to taste

1 ½ cup frozen spinach, defrosted

¼ cup pitted olives, chopped

3 tbsp coconut flour

¼ cup water

1 ½ cups vegan barbecue sauce

1 (14 oz) cranberry sauce

1 tbsp cornstarch + 1 tbsp water

Instructions:

In a food processor, add the tofu, onion, garlic, oregano, salt, black pepper, spinach, olives, and coconut flour. Combine the ingredients evenly. After, make bite-size balls out of the mixture and place on a plate.

Open the instant pot, pour in the water, barbecue sauce, and cranberry sauce. Mix well.

Put the tofu balls into the pot, close the lid, secure the pressure valve, and select Manual mode on high pressure. Cook for 5 minutes.

When the timer has read to the end, do a natural pressure release for 5 minutes, then a quick pressure release, and open the lid.

Combine the cornstarch with the water and pour over the balls and sauce.

Select Sauté mode and allow the sauce to thicken for 2 to 5 minutes.

Turn the pot off after and spoon the tofu balls with cranberry sauce into serving bowls. Allow cooling for a few minutes and serve after.

Nutrition:

Calories 482, Carbohydrates 75.4 g, Fats 11.1 g, Protein 26.7 g

237. Faux Chicken Wings in Barbecue Sauce

Preparation Time: 10 minutes

Cooking Time: 30 minutes

Servings: 4

Ingredients:

For the faux wings:

1 cup wheat gluten

1 tsp onion powder

2 tbsp nutritional yeast

½ tsp salt

½ tsp Italian mixed herbs

3 ¾ cup vegetable broth, divided

2 tbsp tahini

For the barbecue sauce:

½ cup ketchup

1 tbsp coconut sugar

1 tbsp freshly squeezed lemon juice

3 tbsp apple cider vinegar

½ tsp smoked paprika

½ tsp onion powder

½ tsp garlic powder

½ tsp chili powder

1 tbsp mustard

1/3 cup water

Instructions:

In a medium bowl, mix the wheat gluten, onion powder, nutritional yeast, salt, and mixed herbs.

Then, in a smaller bowl, combine the ¾ cup of vegetable broth with the tahini until properly mixed. Add the wet ingredients to the dry ones and combine until a dough forms.

Place the dough on a clean flat surface and knead until elastic but not dry. After, cut the dough into small rounds and try sharpening into chicken wing shapes. Note that the dough will rise 2 to 3 times more after a while, so keep the wing sizes small.

Turn on, open the instant pot, and pour in the remaining broth. Drop the faux wings in the pot, close the lid, secure the pressure valve, and select Manual mode on high pressure. Cook for 10 minutes.

When the timer is done, perform a natural pressure release for 10 minutes, then a quick pressure release, and then open the lid.

Fetch out the wings with broth into a casserole dish and broil in an oven, turning once until both sides are golden brown, 5 to 10 minutes.

Clean the inner part of the instant pot to make the barbecue sauce. In the pot, combine the ketchup, coconut sugar, lemon juice, apple cider vinegar, smoked paprika, onion powder, garlic powder, chili powder, mustard, and water. Stir to mix properly.

Close the lid, secure the pressure valve to sealing, and select Manual mode on high pressure. Cook for 5 minutes.

When the timer is done, perform a quick pressure release, and open the lid.

Pour the faux wings into the sauce and toss to coat on all sides.

Return the wings to the casserole dish and broil further in the oven for 5 minutes.

Take out the wings and serve warm.

Nutrition:

Calories 224, Carbohydrates 40.7 g, Fats 5.1 g, Protein 8.2 g

238. Spicy Corn Fritters with Avocado Sauce

Preparation Time: 20 minutes

Cooking Time: 15 minutes

Servings: 6

Ingredients:

For the corn fritters:

2 ½ cups canned yellow corn, drained

2 tbsp sunflower oil + extra for frying

3 garlic cloves, crushed

2 tbsp ginger powder

Salt and black pepper to taste

2 tbsp chopped parsley

1 fresh red chili, deseeded and minced

½ cup freshly chopped oregano

¼ cup water

Plain flour for dusting

For the avocado sauce:

2 ripe avocados, pitted

2 tomatoes, ripe

½ lemon, juiced

3 garlic cloves, crushed

6 green onions

1 tsp maple syrup

3 tbsp canned pinto beans

1 celery stick, chopped

1 tbsp freshly chopped parsley

Instructions:

In a food processor, add the corn, 2 tablespoons of sunflower oil, garlic, ginger, salt, black pepper, parsley, red chili, oregano, and water. Blend the ingredients until evenly combined.

After, form 2-inch patties out of the batter using your hands, place on a paper towel-lined plate, and refrigerate for 20 minutes.

Turn on, open the instant pot and add 3 tbsp of sunflower oil. Select Sauté mode to heat the oil. When ready, dust the patties with a little flour and fry in batches until golden brown on both sides, 15 minutes.

Remove the patties onto a wire rack to drain the oil while you make the avocado sauce.

In a blender, add the avocados' pulp, tomatoes, lemon juice, garlic, green onions, maple syrup, pinto beans, celery stick, and parsley. Process the ingredients until smooth and pour into a serving bowl.

Nutrition:

Calories 553, Carbohydrates 83 g, Fats 22.6 g, Protein 12.9 g

239. Olives & Vegan Cheese Scones

Preparation Time: 10 minutes

Cooking Time: 20 minutes

Servings: 4

Ingredients:

1 lb. whole meal flour, sifted

2 tbsp baking powder

A pinch salt

A pinch cayenne peppers

2 oz vegan butter

1 cup grated vegan cheese

1 ¼ cup almond milk

¼ cup chopped pitted Kalamata olives

Instructions:

In a medium bowl, mix the flour, baking powder, salt, and cayenne pepper. Add the vegan butter and mix until the mixture looks like fine crumbs.

Whisk in the vegan cheese, olives, and a little milk to combine the dough and soft enough to handle. Transfer to a clean, flat surface and knead into a 1-inch thickness. Cut out 3 to 5 rounds from the dough and form into 3-inch rounds.

Turn on, open the instant pot, and pour in the water. Fit a trivet into the pot and place the scones on top. Close the lid, secure the pressure valve, and select Manual mode on high pressure. Set the timer for 20 minutes.

Once done baking, do a natural pressure release for 10 minutes, and open the lid. Remove the scones onto a wire rack to cool before serving.

Nutrition:

Calories 675, Carbohydrates 98 g, Fats 25 g, Protein 20.8 g

240. Steamed Cabbage Dumplings

Preparation Time: 20 minutes

Cooking Time: 16 minutes

Servings: 4

Ingredients:

2 tsp sesame oil

1 cup minced white mushrooms

½ cup grated carrot

½ shredded red cabbage

1 tbsp rice vinegar

2 tbsp tamari sauce

1 tsp grated ginger

12 vegan dumpling wrappers

Olive oil for coating

2 cups of water

Instructions:

Turn on, open the instant pot, and select Sauté mode. Add the sesame oil to heat and put in the mushrooms. Cook with occasional stirring until the mushrooms soften, 5 minutes.

Top with the carrot, cabbage, rice vinegar, tamari sauce, and ginger. Stir-fry the ingredients until dry, 4 minutes. Turn the heat off.

Place a small bowl of water next to you and lay a dumpling wrapper on a cutting board. Spoon a tablespoon of the sautéed vegetables into the middle side of the wrapper, fold the wrapper over the filling into a half moon, and press together. Repeat this process for the remaining wrappers.

Brush a steamer basket with olive oil and place in the dumplings.

Clean up the instant pot and pour in the water. Fit in the steamer basket and close the lid. Secure the pressure valve, select Steam mode, and set the timer to 7 minutes. Perform a quick pressure release, and open the lid.

Remove the dumplings onto a plate using tongs, allow cooling for a few minutes, and serve with chili dipping sauce.

Nutrition:

Calories 186, Carbohydrates 7.5 g, Fats 15.9 g, Protein 4.5 g

241. Mushrooms in Mini Lettuce Wraps

Preparation Time: 20 minutes

Cooking Time: 15 minutes

Servings: 4

Ingredients:

2 garlic cloves, minced

1 medium white onion, chopped

1 tbsp grated ginger

¼ cup tamari sauce

2 tbsp sesame oil

¼ cup coconut sugar

2 tbsp rice wine vinegar

2 tbsp chili sauce

¼ cup vegetable broth

1 lb Portobello mushrooms, chopped

1 tbsp cornstarch mixed with 2 tbsp water

1 tsp sesame seeds

1 tbsp chopped scallions

1 head endive lettuce, leaves extracted

Lime wedges for serving

Instructions:

Turn on and open the instant pot.

Pour in the garlic, onion, ginger, tamari sauce, sesame oil, coconut sugar, rice wine vinegar, chili sauce, and vegetable broth. Stir to combine and add the mushrooms. Mix again and allow sitting for 15 minutes.

Close the lid, secure the pressure valve, and select Manual mode on high pressure. Cook for 20 minutes.

When the timer is done, perform a natural pressure release for 10 minutes, then a quick pressure release to let out the remaining steam, and open the lid.

Select Sauté mode and add the cornstarch. Cook until the sauce thickens, five minutes and stir in the sesame seeds and scallions. Turn the heat off.

Now, lay 2 lettuce leaves on each other and spoon 1 to 2 tablespoons of the mushrooms filling onto the middle. Serve warm with the lime wedges.

Nutrition:

Calories 482, Carbohydrates 96 g, Fats 8.7 g, Protein 14.9 g

242. Chocolate Chip Cookie in a Jar

Preparation Time: 5 minutes

Cooking Time: 7 minutes

Servings: 4

Ingredients:

½ cup vegan butter, melted

½ cup beet sugar

½ cup coconut sugar

1 tsp vanilla extract

1 cup all-purpose flour

1 tsp baking soda

¼ tsp salt

1 tbsp almond milk

3 ½ oz vegan dark chocolate

Vegan dark chocolate for topping

Instructions:

In a medium bowl, mix the vegan butter, beet sugar, coconut sugar, and vanilla extract. Then, whisk in the flour, baking soda, and salt until evenly combined. Add the almond milk, mix, and fold in the vegan dark chocolate.

Pour the mixture into 4 medium mason jars, and cover with aluminum foil.

Open the instant pot and pour in 2 cups of water. Fit in a trivet and sit the mason jars on top.

Close the lid, secure the pressure valve, and select Manual mode on high pressure. Set the timer for 7 minutes.

When ready, perform a quick pressure release until all the steam has escaped, and open the lid.

Remove the jars onto a flat surface, take off the aluminum foil, and top with some extra chocolate.

Allow cooling for a few minutes and serve.

Nutrition:

Calories 523, Carbohydrates 56 g, Fats 30.9 g, Protein 5.8 g

243. Mixed Fruit Flap Jacks

Preparation Time: 5 minutes

Cooking Time: 2 minutes

Servings: 6

Ingredients:

½ cup vegan butter

2 cups peanut butter

½ cup maple syrup

1 cup rolled oats

1 cup chopped almonds and pecans

¼ cup raisins

¼ cup dried dates

3 tbsp dried goji berries

Instructions:

Turn on, open the instant pot, and select Sauté mode.

Add the vegan butter, peanut butter, and maple syrup, melt all three while stirring continuously, about 2 minutes.

Stir in the rolled oats, almonds, pecans, raisins, dates, and goji berries. Turn the pot off when properly combined.

Allow cooling for 5 to 10 minutes and spoon the mixture onto a baking tray. Use your hands to form a ½-inch rectangular tray. Refrigerate for 2 hours.

After, cut into squares and serve.

Nutrition:

Calories 687, Carbohydrates 67 g, Fats 45 g, Protein 13.9 g

244. Tangy Applesauce Jar with Raisins

Preparation Time: 5 minutes

Cooking Time: 9 minutes

Servings: 4

Ingredients:

12 red apples, cored and chopped

½ lemon, juiced

1 cup water

4 tbsp raisins

Broken vegan tortilla chips

Instructions:

Open the instant pot and pour in the apples, lemon juice, and water.

Close the lid, secure the pressure valve, and select Manual mode on high pressure. Cook for 9 minutes.

When the timer beeps, do a natural pressure release until all the steam is released, and open the lid.

Mash the ingredients with an immersion blender until almost smooth.

Stir in the raisins, spoon the mixture into 4 medium mason jars, and seal the lids. Freeze for 2 hours.

When ready to serve, open the jars, sprinkle with the tortilla chips and serve.

Nutritional Fact per Serving:

Calories 348, Fat 2.5g, Carbs 87.9g, Protein 2.1g

245. Pumpkin Spice Popcorn

Preparation Time: 5 Minutes

Cooking Time: 7 minutes

Servings: 4

Ingredients:

7 cups corn kernels

6 tbsp vegan butter, divided

½ tsp salt

½ tsp baking soda

1 cup coconut sugar

½ cup maple syrup

1 tbsp coconut oil

1 tsp vanilla extract

2 tsp pumpkin pie spice

Instructions:

Turn on the instant pot and select Sauté mode to preheat the pot.

When the display section reads HOT, add half of the vegan butter to melt.

Pour the corn kernels into the pot and cover the pot with a glass lid that fits well.

Allow corns to pop, about 5 minutes. After, turn off the pot and transfer the popcorns to a bowl.

Select Sauté mode on the pot and add the remaining vegan butter to melt.

Meanwhile, in a small bowl, quickly mix the salt, baking soda, coconut sugar, maple syrup, coconut oil, vanilla, and pumpkin pie spice. Pour the mixture into the pot and allow simmering for 1 to 2 minutes. Turn the heat off after and allow cooling.

Pour the popcorn into the pot when the sauce is almost completely cooled and mix to coat with the sauce.

Transfer to serving bowls and enjoy.

Nutritional Fact per Serving:

Calories 591, Total Fat 24.7g, Total Carbs 95.3g, Protein 6.9g

246. Classic Potato Fries

Preparation Time: 5 minutes., Cook Time: 15 minutes

Servings: 8

Ingredients:

2 pounds russet potatoes, peeled and slice to make fries

1/2 teaspoon baking soda

2 teaspoons kosher salt

Canola oil to deep fry as needed

2 cups cold water

Instructions:

Take Instant Pot and carefully arrange it over a clean, dry kitchen platform. Turn on the appliance.

Pour the water, soda and, salt in the cooking pot area. Arrange the trivet inside it; arrange the potatoes over the trivet.

Close the pot lid and seal the valve to avoid any leakage. Find and press "Manual" cooking setting and set cooking time to 2 minutes.

Allow the recipe ingredients to cook for the set time, and after that, the timer reads "zero".

Press "Cancel" and press "NPR" setting for natural pressure release. It takes 8-10 times for all inside pressure to release.

Open the pot and take out the fries.

Take a deep-frying pan and add in the oil to a half depth of the pan size. Heat the pan over medium heat.

Add the fries in batches and fry until it is light golden brown. Enjoy the fries!

Nutrition:

Calories 168, Carbohydrates 38 g, Fats 0 g, Protein 5 g

247. Soy Sauce Tofu

Preparation Time: 10 minutes

Cooking Time: 2 hours 30 minutes

Servings: 2

Ingredients:

1/2 tablespoon apple cider vinegar

1 tablespoon soy sauce

1/4 teaspoon garlic powder

1/4 teaspoon salt

1 container extra firm tofu, prepare 1-inch cubes

1/2 tablespoon red pepper flakes

3/4 cup ketchup

1 1/2 tablespoon brown sugar

Instructions:

Take Instant Pot and carefully arrange it over a clean, dry kitchen platform. Turn on the appliance.

In the cooking pot area, add the mentioned ingredients. Stir the ingredients gently.

Close the pot lid and seal the valve to avoid any leakage. Find and press "Slow cook" cooking setting and set cooking time to 2 hours 30 minutes.

Allow the recipe ingredients to cook for the set time, and after that, the timer reads "zero".

Press "Cancel" and press "NPR" setting for natural pressure release. It takes 8-10 times for all inside pressure to release.

Cook for more time in the mix is too watery.

Open the pot and arrange the cooked recipe in serving plates. Enjoy the vegan recipe!

Nutrition:

Calories 246, Carbohydrates 21 g, Fats 4 g, Protein 11.5 g

Chapter 8. Side dishes

248. Peppers Rice

Preparation time: 10 minutes

Cooking time: 25 minutes

Servings: 4

Ingredients:

1 yellow bell pepper, chopped

1 red bell pepper, chopped

1 green bell pepper, chopped

4 scallions, chopped

2 cups cauliflower rice

1 cup vegetable stock

1 tablespoon olive oil

1 teaspoon coriander, ground

1 teaspoon cumin, ground

1 teaspoon basil, dried

1 teaspoon oregano, dried

A pinch of salt and black pepper

1 tablespoon chives, chopped

Directions:

Heat up a pan with the oil over medium heat, add the scallions and the peppers and sauté for 5 minutes.

Add the cauliflower rice and the other ingredients, toss, cook over medium heat for 20 minutes, divide between plates and serve as a side dish.

Nutrition: calories 69, fat 4.4, fiber 1.3, carbs 8.9, protein 1.3

249. Cauliflower and Chives Mash

Preparation time: 10 minutes

Cooking time: 20 minutes

Servings: 4

Ingredients:

2 pounds cauliflower florets

2 cups water

1 teaspoon thyme, dried

1 teaspoon cumin, dried

1 cup coconut cream

2 garlic cloves, minced

A pinch of salt and black pepper

Directions:

Put the cauliflower florets in a pot, add the water and the other ingredients except the cream, bring to a simmer and cook over medium heat for 20 minutes.

Drain the cauliflower, add the cream, mash everything with a potato masher, whisk well, divide between plates and serve.

Nutrition: calories 200, fat 14.7, fiber 7.2, carbs 16.3, protein 6.1

250. Baked Artichokes and Green Beans

Preparation time: 10 minutes

Cooking time: 40 minutes

Servings: 4

Ingredients:

1 pound green beans, trimmed and halved

3 scallions, chopped

2 tablespoons olive oil

1 cup canned artichoke hearts, drained and quartered

2 garlic cloves, minced

1/3 cup tomato passata

A pinch of salt and black pepper

2 teaspoons mustard powder

1 teaspoon cumin, ground

1 teaspoon coriander, ground

Directions:

Heat up a pan with the oil over medium heat, add the scallions and the garlic and sauté for 5 minutes.

Add the green beans and the other ingredients, toss, introduce in the oven and bake at 390 degrees F for 35 minutes.

Divide the mix between plates and serve as a side dish.

Nutrition: calories 132, fat 7.8, fiber 6.9, carbs 14.8, protein 4.4

251. Cumin Cauliflower Rice and Broccoli

Preparation time: 10 minutes

Cooking time: 25 minutes

Servings: 4

Ingredients:

2 cups cauliflower rice

1 cup broccoli florets

2 tablespoons olive oil

4 scallions, chopped

1 teaspoon sweet paprika

1 teaspoon chili powder

1 cup vegetable stock

1 teaspoon red pepper flakes

A pinch of salt and black pepper

¼ teaspoon cumin, ground

Directions:

Heat up a pan with the oil over medium heat, add the scallions, paprika and chili powder and sauté for 5 minutes.

Add the cauliflower rice and the other ingredients, toss, bring to a simmer, cook over medium heat for 20 minutes, divide between plates and serve.

Nutrition: calories 81, fat 7.9, fiber 1.5, carbs 4.1, protein 1.1

252. Turmeric Cauliflower Rice and Tomatoes

Preparation time: 10 minutes

Cooking time: 25 minutes

Servings: 4

Ingredients:

2 tablespoons olive oil

2 cups cauliflower rice

2 scallions, chopped

2 garlic cloves, minced

1 cup cherry tomatoes, halved

1 teaspoon basil, dried

1 teaspoon oregano, dried

A pinch of salt and black pepper

¼ teaspoon turmeric powder

1 cup vegetable stock

A handful cilantro, chopped

Directions:

Heat up a pan with the oil over medium heat, add the scallions, garlic, basil, oregano and turmeric and sauté for 5 minutes.

Add the cauliflower rice, tomatoes and the remaining ingredients, toss, cook over medium heat for 20 minutes, divide between plates and serve as a side dish.

Nutrition: calories 77, fat 7.7, fiber 1, carbs 3.7, protein 0.7

253. Flavored Tomato and Okra Mix

Preparation time: 10 minutes

Cooking time: 30 minutes

Servings: 6

Ingredients:

1 cup scallions, chopped

1 pound cherry tomatoes, halved

2 cups okra, sliced

2 tablespoons avocado oil

4 garlic cloves, chopped

2 teaspoons oregano, dried

A pinch of salt and black pepper

2 teaspoons cumin, ground

1 cup veggie stock

2 tablespoons tomato passata

Directions:

Heat up a pan with the oil over medium heat, add the scallions and the garlic and sauté for 5 minutes.

Add the tomatoes, the okra and the other ingredients, toss, cook over medium heat for 25 minutes, divide between plates and serve as a side dish.

Nutrition: calories 84, fat 2.1, fiber 5.4, carbs 14.8, protein 4

254. Orange Scallions and Brussels Sprouts

Preparation time: 10 minutes

Cooking time: 25 minutes

Servings: 4

Ingredients:

1 pound Brussels sprouts, trimmed and halved

1 cup scallions, chopped

Zest of 1 lime, grated

1 tablespoon olive oil

¼ cup orange juice

2 tablespoons stevia

A pinch of salt and black pepper

Directions:

Heat up a pan with the oil over medium heat, add the scallions and sauté for 5 minutes.

Add the sprouts and the other ingredients, toss, cook over medium heat for 20 minutes more, divide the mix between plates and serve.

Nutrition: calories 193, fat 4, fiber 1, carbs 8, protein 10

255. Roasted Artichokes and Sauce

Preparation time: 10 minutes

Cooking time: 30 minutes

Servings: 4

Ingredients:

2 big artichokes, trimmed and halved

2 tablespoons avocado oil

Juice of 1 lime

1 teaspoon turmeric powder

1 cup coconut cream

A pinch of salt and black pepper

½ teaspoon onion powder

¼ teaspoon sweet paprika

1 teaspoon cumin, ground

Directions:

In a roasting pan, combine the artichokes with the oil, the lime juice and the other ingredients, toss and bake at 390 degrees F for 30 minutes.

Divide the artichokes and sauce between plates and serve.

Nutrition: calories 190, fat 6, fiber 8, carbs 10, protein 9

256. Zucchini Risotto

Preparation time: 10 minutes

Cooking time: 30 minutes

Servings: 4

Ingredients:

½ cup shallots, chopped

2 tablespoons olive oil

3 garlic cloves, minced

2 cups cauliflower rice

1 cup zucchinis, cubed

2 cups veggie stock

½ cup white mushrooms, chopped

½ teaspoon coriander, ground

A pinch of salt and black pepper

¼ teaspoon oregano, dried

2 tablespoons parsley, chopped

Directions:

Heat up a pan with the oil over medium heat, add the shallots, garlic, mushrooms, coriander and oregano, stir and sauté for 10 minutes.

Add the cauliflower rice and the other ingredients, toss, cook for 20 minutes more, divide between plates and serve.

Nutrition: calories 231, fat 5, fiber 3, carbs 9, protein 12

257. Cabbage and Rice

Preparation time: 10 minutes

Cooking time: 30 minutes

Servings: 4

Ingredients:

1 cup green cabbage, shredded

1 cup cauliflower rice

2 tablespoons olive oil

2 tablespoons tomato passata

2 spring onions, chopped

2 teaspoons balsamic vinegar

A pinch of salt and black pepper

2 teaspoons fennel seeds, crushed

1 teaspoon coriander, ground

Directions:

Heat up a pan with the oil over medium heat, add the spring onions, fennel and coriander, stir and cook for 5 minutes.

Add the cabbage, cauliflower rice and the other ingredients, toss, cook over medium heat for 25 minutes more, divide between plates and serve.

Nutrition: calories 200, fat 4, fiber 1, carbs 8, protein 5

258. Tomato Risotto

Preparation time: 10 minutes

Cooking time: 30 minutes

Servings: 4

Ingredients:

1 cup shallots, chopped

2 cups cauliflower rice

3 tablespoons olive oil

2 cups veggie stock

1 cup tomatoes, crushed

¼ cup cilantro, chopped

½ teaspoon chili powder

1 teaspoon cumin, ground

1 teaspoon coriander, ground

Directions:

Heat up a pan with the oil over medium heat, add the shallots and sauté for 5 minutes.

Add the cauliflower rice, tomatoes and the other ingredients, toss, cook over medium heat for 25 minutes more, divide between plates and serve.

Nutrition: calories 200, fat 4, fiber 3, carbs 6, protein 8

259. Herbed Risotto

Preparation time: 10 minutes

Cooking time: 25 minutes

Servings: 4

Ingredients:

2 cups cauliflower rice

4 scallions, chopped

2 tablespoons avocado oil

2 cups veggie stock

Juice of 1 lime

1 tablespoon parsley, chopped

1 tablespoon cilantro, chopped

1 tablespoon basil, chopped

1 tablespoon oregano, chopped

1 teaspoon sweet paprika

A pinch of salt and black pepper

Directions:

Heat up a pan with the oil over medium heat, add the scallions and sauté for 5 minutes.

Add the cauliflower rice, the stock and the other ingredients, toss, cook over medium heat for 20 minutes, divide between plates and serve as a side dish.

Nutrition: calories 182, fat 4, fiber 2, carbs 8, protein 10

260. Radish and Broccoli

Preparation time: 10 minutes

Cooking time: 30 minutes

Servings: 4

Ingredients:

2 tablespoons olive oil

1 pound broccoli florets

4 scallions, chopped

½ pound radishes, halved

4 garlic cloves, minced

2 teaspoons cumin, ground

2 tablespoons tomato passata

½ cup veggie stock

A pinch of salt and black pepper

Directions:

Heat up a pan with the oil over medium heat, add the scallions and sauté for 5 minutes.

Add the broccoli, radishes and the other ingredients, toss, cook over medium heat for 25 minutes more, divide between plates and serve.

Nutrition: calories 261, fat 5, fiber 4, carbs 9, protein 12

261. Mushrooms and Radishes Mix

Preparation time: 10 minutes

Cooking time: 25 minutes

Servings: 4

Ingredients:

1 pound white mushrooms, halved

½ pound radishes, halved

4 scallions, chopped

4 garlic cloves, minced

2 tablespoons olive oil

½ cup veggie stock

2 tablespoons parsley, chopped

1 teaspoon coriander, ground

1 teaspoon rosemary, dried

A pinch of salt and black pepper

Directions:

Heat up a pan with the oil over medium heat, add the scallions, garlic, coriander and rosemary, stir and cook for 5 minutes.

Add the mushrooms, radishes and the other ingredients, toss, cook over medium heat for 20 minutes, divide between plates and serve as a side dish.

Nutrition: calories 182, fat 4, fiber 2, carbs 6, protein 8

262. Sesame and Chives Rice

Preparation time: 10 minutes

Cooking time: 25 minutes

Servings: 4

Ingredients:

2 tablespoons olive oil

1 cup cauliflower rice

1 cup veggie stock

2 tablespoon shallots, chopped

2 tablespoons chives, chopped

1 teaspoon sesame seeds, toasted

A pinch of salt and black pepper

Directions:

Heat up a pan with the oil over medium heat, add the shallots and chives and sauté for 5 minutes.

Add the cauliflower rice and the other ingredients, toss, cook over medium heat for 20 minutes more, divide between plates and serve.

Nutrition: calories 261, fat 6, fiber 8, carbs 10, protein 6

263. Mashed Broccoli

Preparation time: 10 minutes

Cooking time: 25 minutes

Servings: 4

Ingredients:

1 and ½ cups water

1 pound broccoli florets

2 teaspoons olive oil

A pinch of salt and black pepper

½ teaspoon turmeric powder

½ teaspoon cumin, ground

1 tablespoon chives, chopped

Directions:

Put the water in a pot, add the broccoli, salt and pepper, bring to a boil and cook over medium heat for 25 minutes.

Drain the broccoli, transfer to a bowl, and mash using a potato masher.

Add the rest of the ingredients, mash everything again, stir as well, divide between plates and serve as a side dish.

Nutrition: calories 200, fat 4, fiber 4, carbs 7, protein 10

264. Balsamic Hot Radishes

Preparation time: 10 minutes

Cooking time: 20 minutes

Servings: 4

Ingredients:

2 tablespoons avocado oil

1 pound radishes, halved

1 tablespoon balsamic vinegar

A pinch of salt and black pepper

A pinch of chili powder

Directions:

Heat up a pan with the oil over medium heat, add the radishes, vinegar and the other ingredients, toss, cook for 20 minutes, divide between plates and serve as a side dish.

Nutrition: calories 182, fat 5, fiber 5, carbs 9, protein 9

265. Turmeric Coconut Rice Mix

Preparation time: 10 minutes

Cooking time: 20 minutes

Servings: 4

Ingredients:

1 cup cauliflower rice

1 tablespoon coconut cream

1 cup coconut milk

A pinch of salt and black pepper

1 teaspoon turmeric powder

½ teaspoon garam masala

1 tablespoon cilantro, chopped

Directions:

Put the coconut milk in a pan, heat up over medium heat, add the rice, cream and the other ingredients, toss, cook for 20 minutes, divide between plates and serve.

Nutrition: calories 211, fat 5, fiber 4, carbs 6, protein 12

266. Wild Mushrooms and Radish Rice

Preparation time: 10 minutes

Cooking time: 25 minutes

Servings: 4

Ingredients:

2 cups cauliflower rice

2 tablespoons avocado oil

½ cup wild mushrooms, sliced

½ cup radishes, halved

3 shallots, chopped

1 cup veggie stock

1 teaspoon fennel seeds

1 teaspoon coriander, ground

A pinch of salt and black pepper

2 tablespoons chives, chopped

Directions:

Heat up a pan with the oil over medium heat, add the shallots and the mushrooms and sauté for 5 minutes.

Add the cauliflower rice, the radishes and the other ingredients, toss, cook over medium heat for 20 minutes, divide between plates and serve as a side dish.

Nutrition: calories 189, fat 3, fiber 4, carbs 9, protein 8

267. Hot Okra

Preparation time: 10 minutes

Cooking time: 20 minutes

Servings: 4

Ingredients:

1 pound okra, halved

2 tablespoons avocado oil

4 scallions, chopped

2 garlic cloves, minced

1 tablespoon chili powder

1 teaspoon hot paprika

1 tablespoon balsamic vinegar

A pinch of salt and black pepper

Directions:

Heat up a pan with the oil over medium heat, add the scallions and the garlic and sauté for 5 minutes.

Add the okra and the other ingredients, toss, cook over medium heat for 15 minutes, divide between plates and serve as a side dish.

Nutrition: calories 182, fat 4, fiber 2, carbs 6, protein 6

268. Pineapple Rice

Preparation Time: 5 Minutes

Cooking Time: 8 minutes

Servings: 4

Ingredients:

1 ½ cup of rice

2 cups of water

1 cup pineapple juice

1 can pineapples, chopped

1 teaspoon coconut cream

Instructions:

Pour water and pineapple juice in the instant pot. Add rice and chopped pineapple, and close the lid.

Set Manual mode (high pressure) for 8 minutes. Then use quick pressure release.

Transfer the cooked pineapple rice in the bowl and add coconut cream. Stir it.

Nutrition:

Calories 310, Carbohydrates 69 g, Fats 0.9 g, Protein 5.4 g

269. Mongolian Stir Fry

Preparation Time: 5 Minutes

Cooking Time: 4 minutes

Servings: 4

Ingredients:

1 tablespoon minced ginger

1 teaspoon minced garlic

1 tablespoon avocado oil

4 tablespoons soy sauce

1 teaspoon chili flakes

1 teaspoon cornstarch

1 tablespoon brown sugar

8 tablespoon water

½ teaspoon cayenne pepper

1-pound seitan, chopped

Instructions:

In the mixing bowl whisk together minced ginger, minced garlic, avocado oil, soy sauce, chili flakes, cornstarch, brown sugar, cayenne pepper, and water.

Preheat instant pot bowl on Sauté mode until hot.

Transfer ginger mixture in the instant pot and cook it for 1 minute.

Then add chopped seitan and stir well.

Close the lid and set Manual mode (high pressure) for 1 minute. Use quick pressure release.

Mix up the side dish well before serving.

Nutrition:

Calories 59, Carbohydrates 5.6 g, Fats 0.9 g, Protein 6.6 g

270. Mushroom "Bacon"

Preparation Time: 5 Minutes

Cooking Time: 2 minutes

Servings: 5

Ingredients:

6 oz shiitake mushrooms

1 teaspoon salt

¼ teaspoon cayenne pepper

1 tablespoon olive oil

Instructions:

Slice the mushrooms onto bacon shape strips and sprinkle every strip with olive oil, cayenne pepper, and salt.

Then place mushroom "bacon" in the instant pot and close the lid.

Set Manual mode (high pressure) and cook mushrooms for 2 minutes. Then use quick pressure release. The time of cooking depends on mushroom strips size.

Nutrition:

Calories 43, Carbohydrates 4.7 g, Fats 2.9 g, Protein 0.5 g

271. Crushed Baby Potatoes

Preparation Time: 10 Minutes

Cooking Time: 10 minutes

Servings: 2

Ingredients:

1 ½ cup baby potatoes

1 teaspoon salt

4 tablespoons olive oil

1 tablespoon dried rosemary

1 teaspoon dried oregano

Instructions:

Wash baby potatoes carefully and crush with the help of the knife.

Then sprinkle the crushed potatoes with salt, olive oil, dried rosemary, and oregano.

Shake well until homogenous.

Transfer potatoes in the instant pot and close the lid.

Cook the meal on Manual mode (high pressure) for 4 minutes.

Then use natural pressure release for 5 minutes. Don't mix up potatoes anymore.

Nutrition:

Calories 325, Carbohydrates 19.2 g, Fats 28.4 g, Protein 2.1 g

272. Bang Bang Broccoli

Preparation Time: 10 Minutes

Cooking Time: 4 minutes

Servings: 2

Ingredients:

2 tablespoons vegan mayo

1 teaspoon chili paste

1 tablespoon Maple syrup

1 cup broccoli

¼ cup almond milk

1 teaspoon cornstarch

2 tablespoons wheat flour

1 teaspoon olive oil

1/3 cup panko bread crumbs

1 tablespoon lemon juice

½ cup water for cooking

Instructions:

For the sauce: whisk together vegan mayo and chili paste.

For the broccoli batter: in the separated bowl whisk together almond milk, wheat flour, olive oil, cornstarch, and lemon juice.

Cut broccoli into the florets and dip into the batter.

Then coat every broccoli floret in the panko bread crumbs.

Pour water in the instant pot bowl and insert rack.

Place coated broccoli on the rack and close the lid.

Cook the vegetables on Manual mode (High pressure) for 4 minutes. Use quick pressure release.

Transfer the cooked broccoli in the bowl and sprinkle with sauce.

Nutrition:

Calories 280, Carbohydrates 33.7 g, Fats 14.7 g, Protein 5.4 g

273. Tikka Masala with Cauliflower

Preparation Time: 10 Minutes

Cooking Time: 10 minutes

Servings: 4

Ingredients:

1 teaspoon garam masala

½ teaspoon salt

1 cup cauliflower, chopped

1/3 cup coconut yogurt

1 teaspoon ground cumin

½ teaspoon ground coriander

1 onion, diced

½ teaspoon garlic, diced

¼ teaspoon minced ginger

1 cup tomatoes, canned

Instructions:

Set instant pot on Sauté mode.

Add olive oil, diced onion, garlic, and minced ginger.

Then sprinkle the mixture with ground cumin, coriander, salt, and garam masala.

Mix up well.

Add canned tomatoes and mix up well. Sauté the mixture for 5 minutes.

After this, add chopped cauliflower and stir well.

Close the lid and seal it. Cook the meal on Manual mode (High pressure) for 3 minutes.

Then use quick pressure release and open the lid.

Add coconut yogurt and mix up well. Serve the meal hot

Nutrition:

Calories 67, Carbohydrates 7.2 g, Fats 4.1 g, Protein 1.7 g

274. Vegetable En Papillote

Preparation Time: 10 Minutes

Cooking Time: 3 minutes

Servings: 4

Ingredients:

1 cup baby carrot

½ cup green beans

1 teaspoon dried rosemary

1 teaspoon salt

1 tablespoon avocado oil

1 garlic clove, diced

1 teaspoon fresh oregano

1 tablespoon lemon juice

1 teaspoon turmeric

Instructions:

In the mixing bowl mix up together baby carrot and green beans.

Sprinkle the vegetables with dried rosemary, salt, avocado oil, garlic, oregano, lemon juice, and turmeric. Shake the ingredients well.

Then Wrap the vegetables in the baking paper and transfer in the instant pot.

Close the lid and seal it.

Cook the vegetables on Manual mode (High pressure) for 3 minutes.

Then allow natural pressure release for 5 minutes and remove vegetables from the baking paper.

Nutrition:

Calories 30, Carbohydrates 5.8 g, Fats 0.7 g, Protein 0.7 g

275. Brown Rice

Preparation Time: 15 Minutes

Cooking Time: 18 minutes

Servings: 4

Ingredients:

1 ½ cup brown rice

3 cups of water

1 tablespoon olive oil

1 teaspoon salt

Instructions:

Set Sauté mode and preheat instant pot.

Add olive oil and brown rice and stir it well.

Cook the rice for 3 minutes.

Add water and salt. Close and seal the lid.

Set Manual mode (high pressure) and cook the meal for 15 minutes.

Allow natural pressure release for 10 minutes more.

Mix up the rice before serving.

Nutrition:

Calories 57, Carbohydrates 5.3 g, Fats 3.9 g, Protein 0.4 g

276. Fragrant Bulgur

Preparation Time: 5 Minutes

Cooking Time: 19 minutes

Servings: 3

Ingredients:

1 cup bulgur

1 teaspoon tomato paste

2 cups of water

1 teaspoon olive oil

1 teaspoon salt

Instructions:

Preheat instant pot on Sauté mode and add olive oil.

Place bulgur in the oil and stir well. Sauté it for 4 minutes.

Then add tomato paste and salt. Stir well.

Add water and mix up bulgur until you get a homogenous liquid mixture.

Close the lid and set Manual mode (low pressure).

Cook bulgur for 15 minutes.

The bulgur will be cooked when it soaks all the liquid.

Nutrition:

Calories 174, Carbohydrates 35.8 g, Fats 2.2 g, Protein 5.8 g

277. Baked Apples

Preparation Time: 5 Minutes

Cooking Time: 9 minutes

Servings: 6

Ingredients:

4 red apples, chopped

1 teaspoon ground cinnamon

1 tablespoon brown sugar

1 teaspoon maple syrup

¼ cup cashew milk

Instructions:

Place apples in the instant pot and sprinkle with ground cinnamon, brown sugar, and maple syrup.

Close the lid and set Sauté mode. Cook the apples for 5 minutes.

Then add cashew milk and mix up the side dish well.

Cook it for 4 minutes more.

Nutrition:

Calories 88, Carbohydrates 23.1 g, Fats 0.4 g, Protein 0.4 g

278. Scalloped Potatoes

Preparation Time: 15 Minutes

Cooking Time: 4 minutes

Servings: 4

Ingredients:

4 potatoes, peeled, sliced

1 cup almond milk

1 teaspoon nutritional yeast

1 teaspoon dried rosemary

½ teaspoon salt

1 teaspoon garlic powder

1 teaspoon cashew butter

1 teaspoon ground nutmeg

Instructions:

Mix up together nutritional yeast, dried rosemary, salt, garlic powder, and ground nutmeg. Whisk together almond milk and spice mixture.

Grease the instant pot bowl with cashew butter.

Place the sliced potatoes inside instant pot bowl by layers.

Then pour almond milk mixture over the potatoes and close the lid.

Cook scalloped potatoes on Manual mode (High pressure) for 4 minutes. Then allow natural pressure release for 10 minutes.

Sprinkle the cooked meal with your favorite vegan cheese if desired.

Nutrition:

Calories 302, Carbohydrates 38.5 g, Fats 15.5 g, Protein 5.7 g

279. Glazed White Onions

Preparation Time: 5 Minutes

Cooking Time: 20 minutes

Servings: 4

Ingredients:

3 white onions, peeled, sliced

1 tablespoon sugar

½ teaspoon ground black pepper

3 tablespoons coconut oil

½ teaspoon baking soda

Instructions:

Set Sauté mode and preheat instant pot until hot.

Toss coconut oil and melt it.

When the coconut oil is liquid, add sugar, baking soda, and ground black pepper. Stir the mixture gently.

Add sliced onions and mix the ingredients up.

Close the lid and sauté onions for 15 minutes.

When the side dish is cooked it will have a light brown color and tender texture.

Nutrition:

Calories 133, Carbohydrates 10.9 g, Fats 10.3 g, Protein 0.9 g

280. Spicy Garlic

Preparation Time: 10 Minutes

Cooking Time: 10 minutes

Servings: 4

Ingredients:

4 garlic bulbs, trimmed

2 teaspoons olive oil

½ teaspoon salt

¼ teaspoon chili flakes

½ cup water, for cooking

Instructions:

Pour water in the instant pot and insert rack.

Place garlic bulbs on the rack and sprinkle with olive oil, salt, and chili flakes.

Close the lid and set Poultry mode.

Cook garlic for 10 minutes. Then allow natural pressure release for 5 minutes more.

Serve the garlic when it reaches room temperature.

Nutrition:

Calories 35, Carbohydrates 3 g, Fats 2.3 g, Protein 0 g

281. Pasta and Green Peas Side Dish

Preparation Time: 5 Minutes

Cooking Time: 10 minutes

Servings: 2

Ingredients:

½ cup pasta

1 cup of water

1/3 cup green peas, frozen

1 teaspoon salt

¼ teaspoon minced garlic

1 teaspoon tomato paste

Instructions:

Mix up together water, tomato paste, minced garlic, and salt.

Pout liquid in the instant pot. Add green peas and pasta. Mix up gently.

Close the lid and set Manual mode (High pressure).

Cook the side dish for 10 minutes. Then use quick pressure release.

Drain ½ part of the liquid and transfer the meal into the serving bowls

Nutrition:

Calories 207, Carbohydrates 39.1 g, Fats 1.6 g, Protein 8.7 g

282. Almond Milk Millet

Preparation Time: 5 Minutes

Cooking Time: 10 minutes

Servings: 3

Ingredients:

½ teaspoon salt

1 cup millet

1 cup almond milk

Instructions:

Pour almond milk in the instant pot bowl.

Add millet and salt.

Close and seal the lid and set Manual mode (High pressure).

Cook the side dish for 10 minutes. Allow natural pressure release.

Nutrition:

Calories 436, Carbohydrates 53 g, Fats 21.9 g, Protein 9.2 g

283. Stir Fried Kale

Preparation Time: 5 Minutes

Cooking Time: 5 minutes

Servings: 4

Ingredients:

2 cup kale, chopped

½ teaspoon nutritional yeast

1 teaspoon coconut oil

½ teaspoon ground black pepper

2 tablespoons bread crumbs

4 tablespoons water

Instructions:

Preheat instant pot on Sauté mode until hot.

Toss coconut oil and melt it.

Add chopped kale and sprinkle it with ground black pepper and nutritional yeast.

Add water and sauté kale for 2 minutes.

Then mix up kale well and sprinkle with bread crumbs.

Close the lid and cook on Manual mode (high pressure) for 1 minute. Allow quick pressure release.

Shake the kale well before serving.

Nutrition:

Calories 42 , Carbohydrates 6.3 g, Fats 1.3 g, Protein 1.7 g

284. Zoodles

Preparation Time: 10 Minutes

Cooking Time: 25 minutes

Servings: 4

Ingredients:

2 zucchinis

½ teaspoon salt

¾ cup vegetable broth

¼ teaspoon ground black pepper

Instructions:

Wash and trim zucchini well.

With the help of the spiralizer make the zucchini zoodles.

Sprinkle them with ground black pepper and salt.

Transfer zoodles in the instant pot bowl and add vegetable broth.

Close and seal the lid. Set Manual mode (high pressure) and cook meal for 1 minute. Use natural pressure release.

Nutrition:

Calories 23, Carbohydrates 3.5 g, Fats 0.4 g, Protein 2.1 g

285. Buckwheat

Preparation Time: 10 Minutes

Cooking Time: 15 minutes

Servings: 4

Ingredients:

2 cups buckwheat

¼ cup of water

1 tablespoon sunflower oil

1 teaspoon salt

1 tablespoon almond butter

Instructions:

Pour sunflower oil in the instant pot. Add almond butter and sauté the ingredients for 3 minutes on Sauté mode.

Then add buckwheat and stir it carefully. Sauté the mixture for 3 minutes.

Add water and stir well.

Close and seal the lid.

Set manual mode (high pressure) and cook buckwheat for 4 minutes.

Then use quick pressure release.

Mix up the buckwheat carefully before serving.

Nutrition:

Calories 347, Carbohydrates 61.5 g, Fats 8.6 g, Protein 12.1 g

Chapter 9. Dessert

286. Vanilla Pudding

Preparation Time: 25 Minutes

Cooking Time: 10 Minutes

Servings: 2

Ingredients

1 tablespoon maple syrup

1 tablespoon corn starch

1/8 teaspoon salt

2 cups coconut milk

1 large egg yolks

½ tablespoon unsalted butter

1 teaspoon pure vanilla extract

Instructions

In an instant pot combine together maple syrup, corn-starch, salt, coconut milk, and egg yolks. Cover your Instant Pot, set the vent to 'sealing,' select the manual or pressure cook button, select high pressure and set the timer to 05 mins.

When done allow the pot to undergo natural pressure release for 15 mins

About 8-10 minutes. Note: It will thicken more as it cools.

Place a fine mesh strainer over a large heatproof bowl. Pour the mixture through the strainer and into the bowl.

Transfer the pudding from the large bowl or into individual serving bowls. Cool slightly, then cover with plastic wrap. Refrigerate for several hours or until chilled.

Nutrition:

Calories 654, Total Fat 62.4g, Saturated Fat 53.4g, Cholesterol 113mg, Sodium 209mg, Total Carbohydrate 25.1g, Dietary Fiber 5.3g, Total Sugars 14.3g, Protein 6.9g

287. Quick Cherry Crisp

Preparation Time: 25 Minutes

Cooking Time: 25 Minutes

Servings: 2

Ingredients

¼ cup honey

½ tablespoon corn-starch

2 cups red cherries

½ cup crumbled shortbread cookies

1 tablespoon butter or margarine, melted

1/8 cup chopped almonds, toasted

Ice cream (optional)

Instructions

In a small bowl, combine honey and corn-starch. In an instant pot, sprinkle corn-starch mixture over cherries; stir to combine. 1. Cover your Instant Pot, set the vent to 'sealing,' select the manual or pressure cook button, select high pressure and set the timer to 02 mins.

When done allow the pot to undergo natural pressure release for 15 mins 10 minutes or until thickened and bubbly.

Meanwhile, in a medium bowl, thoroughly combine crumbled cookies, butter, and nuts

Divide cherry mixture among four dessert dishes. Sprinkle cookie mixture over cherry mixture. If desired, serve with ice cream.

Nutrition:

Calories223, Total Fat 8.7g, Saturated Fat 3.9g, Cholesterol 15mg , Sodium 43mg, Total Carbohydrate 38.4g, Dietary Fiber 0.8g, Total Sugars 35.1g, Protein 1.5g

288. Chocolate Chip Cheesecake

Preparation Time: 25 Minutes

Cooking Time: 25 Minutes

Servings: 2

Ingredients

½ cup graham cracker crumbs

1 tablespoon honey

½ cup unsweetened cocoa powder

½ cup butter, melted

½ cup cream cheese

1 cup sweetened condensed milk

1 egg

1 teaspoon vanilla extract

½ cup mini semi-sweet chocolate chips

1 teaspoon coconut flour

Instructions

Mix graham cracker crumbs, honey, butter and cocoa. Press onto bottom and up the sides of a 9 inch spring form pan. Set crust aside.

Beat cream cheese until smooth. Gradually add sweetened condensed milk; beat well. Add vanilla and egg, and beat on medium speed until smooth. Toss 1/3 of the miniature chocolate chips with the 1 teaspoon coconut flour to coat (this keeps them from sinking to the bottom of the cake). Mix into cheese mixture. Pour into prepared crust. Sprinkle top with remaining chocolate chips.

Pour the water into the Instant Pot Insert, and place a trivet with the covered brownie cake tin into the Instant Pot.

Cover your Instant Pot, set the vent to 'sealing,' select the manual or pressure cook button, select high pressure and set the timer to 30 mins.

When done allow the pot to undergo natural pressure release for 15 mins

Refrigerate before removing sides of pan. Keep cake refrigerated until time to serve.

Nutrition:

Calories 656, Total Fat 43.3g, Saturated Fat 26.4g, Cholesterol 160mg, Sodium 458mg, Total Carbohydrate 61.5g, Dietary Fiber 4.3g, Total Sugars 48.4g, Protein 12.7g

289. Peanut Butter Fudge

Preparation Time: 25 Minutes

Cooking Time: 25 Minutes

Servings: 2

Ingredients

1 tablespoon honey

1/8 cup coconut milk

½ cup marshmallow crème

1 cups peanut butter

Instructions

In Instant pot Select Sauté Add coconut milk and honey .Cover your Instant Pot, set the vent to 'sealing,' select the manual or pressure cook button, select high pressure and set the timer to 3 mins.

When done allow the pot to undergo natural pressure release for 15 mins

Immediately stir in the marshmallow crème and peanut butter.

Pour and spread into a 9x9 inch glass baking dish. Cool completely before cutting into squares and serving.

Nutrition:

Calories 412, Total Fat 34.2g, Saturated Fat 8.4g, Cholesterol 0mg 0%, Sodium 298mg, Total Carbohydrate 17.5g, Dietary Fiber 4g , Total Sugars 10.6g, Protein 16.3g

290. Banana-Oatmeal Cake

Preparation Time: 15 Minutes

Cooking Time: 35 Minutes

Servings: 2

Ingredients

½ cup coconut milk

1tablespoon honey

2 tablespoons coconut oil

1/4 tablespoon butter, melted

1 teaspoon baking soda

1 teaspoon baking powder

¼ cup oats

½ teaspoon vanilla extract

1 cup coconut flour

¼ cup mashed bananas

Instructions

Lightly grease a 9x13-inch baking dish.

Mix coconut milk and vanilla extract together in a bowl.

Stir honey, coconut oil, coconut milk mixture, and butter together in a bowl; add baking soda and baking powder and stir. Mix oats into honey mixture. Stir coconut flour, 1 cup at a time, into oat mixture until batter is evenly combined; fold in bananas. Pour batter into the prepared baking dish.

Pour the water into the Instant Pot Insert, and place a trivet with the covered brownie cake tin into the Instant Pot.

Cover your Instant Pot, set the vent to 'sealing,' select the manual or pressure cook button, select high pressure and set the timer to 35 mins.

When done allow the pot to undergo natural pressure release for 15 mins

Nutrition:

Calories 194, Total Fat 15.5g, Saturated Fat 13.3g, Cholesterol 2mg, Sodium 334mg, Total Carbohydrate 14.2g, Dietary Fiber 2.7g, Total Sugars 6.8g, Protein 2g

291. Fresh Apple Cake

Preparation Time: 15 Minutes

Cooking Time: 35 Minutes

Servings: 2

Ingredients

1 tablespoon maple syrup

1/8 cup butter

1 egg

1/2 cups flex meal flour

¼ teaspoon baking soda

1 pinch salt

½ teaspoon ground nutmeg

½ teaspoon vanilla extract

½ cup apple - peeled, cored, and chopped

1/8 cup chopped almonds

Instructions

Grease a 9 inch pan. In a medium bowl, mix the flex meal flour, baking soda, salt and nutmeg together and set aside.

In a large bowl, cream the butter and maple syrup until fluffy. Add the egg and beat well. Add the vanilla extract. Add the flour mixture and beat well. Fold in the chopped apples and almonds.

Pour batter into a greased 9 inch pan.

Pour the water into the Instant Pot Insert, and place a trivet with the covered brownie cake tin into the Instant Pot.

Cover your Instant Pot, set the vent to 'sealing,' select the manual or pressure cook button, select high pressure and set the timer to 35 mins.

When done allow the pot to undergo natural pressure release for 15 mins.

Enjoy.

Nutrition:

Calories 174, Total Fat 11g, Saturated Fat 4.2g , Cholesterol 56mg , Sodium 190mg, Total Carbohydrate 13.1g, Dietary Fiber 5.1g , Total Sugars 6.2g, Protein 7.2g

292. Apple Banana Cupcakes

Preparation Time: 15 Minutes

Cooking Time: 25 Minutes

Servings: 2

Ingredients

¼ cup chia seed flour

½ teaspoon baking soda

Pinch salt

2 tablespoon coconut oil

¼ teaspoon ground nutmeg

1/8 teaspoon ground clove

2 tablespoon honey

1 egg

½ teaspoon vanilla extract

1/8 cup buttermilk

¼ cup ripe bananas, mashed

1 apple- peeled, cored and shredded

Instructions

Grease and flour 12 muffin cups, or use paper liners. Sift together the chia seed flour, baking soda, salt, cinnamon, and nutmeg. Set aside.

In a large bowl, cream together the honey and coconut oil until light and fluffy. Beat in the eggs one at a time, then stir in the vanilla extract and buttermilk. Beat in the flour mixture, mixing just until incorporated. Fold in the mashed bananas and shredded apples. Fill each muffin cup half full.

Set trivet into inner pot of the Instant Pot. Add 1 cup water. Set muffins cups on trivet.

Secure lid, ensuring the valve is pointed to sealing. Press pressure cook and set timer to 20 minutes.

When timer goes off, turn valve to venting to release the pressure. When all pressure is released, carefully remove lid and take out dish.

Allow to cool slightly before serving

Nutrition:

Calories99, Total Fat 1.6g, Saturated Fat 0.5g, Cholesterol 41mg , Sodium 238mg, Total Carbohydrate 20.4g, Dietary Fiber 1.8g , Total Sugars 16.2g, Protein 2.1g

293. **Banana Chocolate Chip Cake**

Preparation Time: 15 Minutes

Cooking Time: 25 Minutes

Servings: 2

Ingredients

1 cup Oat flour

2 tablespoons honey

1 teaspoon baking powder

¼ teaspoon salt

¼ cup mashed bananas

1 egg

2 tablespoons vegetable oil

¼ cup coconut milk

¼ cup semisweet chocolate chips

Instructions

Grease and flour a 9x13 inch pan.

In a large bowl, mix oat flour, honey, baking powder and salt.

In a separate bowl, combine bananas, egg, coconut oil and coconut milk.

Stir banana mixture into flour mixture until blended. Be careful not to over mix.

Stir in chocolate chips.

Pour batter into 9x13 inch pan.

Set trivet into inner pot of the Instant Pot. Add 1 cup water. Set muffins cups on trivet.

Secure lid, ensuring the valve is pointed to sealing. Press pressure cook and set timer to 35 minutes.

When timer goes off, turn valve to venting to release the pressure. When all pressure is released, carefully remove lid and take out dish.

Allow to cool slightly before serving

Nutrition:

Calories 624, Total Fat 34g, Saturated Fat 15.5g, Cholesterol 82mg , Sodium 329mg, Total Carbohydrate 74.1g, Dietary Fiber 7.2g, Total Sugars 34.7g, Protein 9.7g

294. Blueberry Buttermilk Coffeecake

Preparation Time: 15 Minutes

Cooking Time: 25 Minutes

Servings: 2

Ingredients

2 cups coconut flour

1 teaspoons baking powder

½ teaspoon baking soda

Pinch salt

2 tablespoon maple syrup

2 tablespoon avocado oil

1 egg

¼ teaspoon vanilla extract

1 cup buttermilk

1 cup blueberries

Instructions

Grease and flour an 8 inch pan.

Sift coconut flour, baking powder, baking soda, and salt together in a bowl. Set aside.

In a large bowl, cream together maple syrup and coconut oil until light and fluffy. Beat in eggs one at a time, then stir in the vanilla. Beat in the flour mixture alternately with the buttermilk, mixing just until incorporated. Sir in blueberries. Pour batter into prepared pan.

Pour water into Instant Pot. Place wire trivet into the bottom of the pot and set the pan on top. Place lid on pot and lock into place to seal. Pressure Cook or Manual on High Pressure for 30 minutes. Let sit 10 minutes. Use Quick Pressure Release.

Nutrition:

Calories171, Total Fat 4.9g, Saturated Fat 2.5g, Cholesterol 58mg, Sodium 391mg, Total Carbohydrate 26.6g, Dietary Fiber 5g, Total Sugars 17.5g, Protein 6.4g

295. Prunes Cake

Preparation Time: 40 Minutes

Cooking Time: 25 Minutes

Servings: 2

Ingredients

¼ cup vegetable oil

¼ cup honey

1 egg

2 cups coconut flour

½ teaspoon salt

1 teaspoon baking powder

1 cup coconut milk

1 teaspoon vanilla extract

¼ teaspoon almond extract

2 cups chopped prunes, divided

¼ cup water

1 tablespoon lemon juice

Instructions

Spray two 8-inch round cake pans with vegetable oil spray.

In a medium bowl, sift together coconut flour, salt and baking powder. Set aside.

In a large mixing bowl, making cream add vegetable oil with the honey until fluffy. Add egg and beat well. Add flour mixture coconut milk. Fold in vanilla and almond extracts and 1 cup chopped prunes.

Pour water into Instant Pot. Place wire trivet into the bottom of the pot and set the pan on top. Place lid on pot and lock into place to seal. Pressure Cook or Manual on High Pressure for 30 minutes. Let sit 10 minutes. Use Quick Pressure Release. Keep cake aside.

To make the filling: In an Instant pot, combine reaming chopped prunes, honey, and water and lemon juice. Close the lid of Instant pot, Pressure Cook or Manual on High Pressure for 20 minutes. Let sit 10 minutes. Use

Quick Pressure Release. Spread thinly between cooled cake layers and on top.

Nutrition:

Calories539, Total Fat 23.9g, Saturated Fat 12.7g, Cholesterol 33mg, Sodium 256mg, Total Carbohydrate 77.2g, Dietary Fiber 4.9g, Total Sugars 28.9g, Protein 8.2g

296. Butternut squash. -Almond Cookies

Preparation Time: 40 Minutes

Cooking Time: 25 Minutes

Servings: 2

Ingredients

1 cup butter, soften

¼ cup honey

1 egg, beaten

¼ teaspoon vanilla extract

1 cup butternut squash. puree

2 cups coconut flour

1 teaspoon baking powder

1 teaspoon baking soda

¼ teaspoon salt

1 teaspoon ground nutmeg

¼ cup walnuts

Instructions

Line the Instant pot with parchment paper and spray with non-stick coconut oil spray. Set aside.

Cream together the butter and honey.

Beat together the egg, vanilla and butternut squash puree.

Sift together the coconut flour, baking powder, baking soda, salt and nutmeg; combine with butternut squash mixture and stir in almond.

Add the cookie dough to the prepared Instant pot. Using a rubber spatula, spread and press the dough into the bottom of the pot, making sure to cover the bottom completely and filling in any gaps.

Cover and lock the lid, but leave the steam release handle in the venting position. Select High pressure and set the cook time for 15 min. When the cook time is complete, press Cancel to turn off the pot.

Open the lid and carefully transfer the inner pot with the cookie to a cooling rack. Allow the cookie to cool in the pot for a minimum of 30 minutes or until it reaches room temperature.

Nutrition:

Calories 187, Total Fat 17.4g, Saturated Fat 10g, Cholesterol 54mg , Sodium 270mg, Total Carbohydrate 8.1g, Dietary Fiber 0.8g , Total Sugars 6.6g, Protein 1.5g

297. Blackberries Compote

Preparation Time: 15 Minutes

Cooking Time: 20 Minutes

Servings: 2

Ingredients

4 cups fresh blackberries

¼ cup maple syrup

1 teaspoon freshly squeezed lemon juice

1 teaspoon orange juice

Instructions

Wash all the blackberries.

Add the blackberries and maple syrup to the Instant pot. Add the lemon juice and orange juice

Lock the lid in place. Select Pressure Cook or Manual, and adjust the pressure to High and the time to 2 minutes. After cooking, let the pressure release naturally for 10 minutes, then quick release any remaining pressure.

Unlock the lid. Taste the berries (carefully—they're hot) and adjust the sweetness if necessary.

Nutrition:

Calories228, Total Fat 1.5g, Saturated Fat 0.1g, Cholesterol 0mg , Sodium 7mg, Total Carbohydrate 54.4g, Dietary Fiber 15.3g , Total Sugars 37.5g, Protein 4g

298. Raspberry-Vanilla Barley Pudding

Preparation Time: 10 Minutes

Cooking Time: 45 Minutes

Servings: 2

Ingredients

1 cup water

1 cup coconut milk

1 tablespoon honey

½ cup raspberries fresh

½ cup barley

¼ teaspoon nutmeg

¼ teaspoon vanilla

½ cup coconut cream

Instructions

Select sauté on the Instant Pot and adjust to normal. Add the coconut milk, water, honey, to the pot.

Press cancel. Stir in the barley and nutmeg and vanilla into the pot. Secure the lid on the Instant pot. Close the pressure-release valve. Select porridge. When cooking is complete, use a natural release to depressurize.

Remove and Stir in fresh raspberries and cream.

Nutrition:

Calories 489,Total Fat 29.9g, Saturated Fat 25.7g, Cholesterol 0mg , Sodium 28mg, Total Carbohydrate 49.3g, Dietary Fiber 10.7g, Total Sugars 13.2g, Protein 8.5g

299. Nectarines Cobbler

Preparation Time: 10 Minutes

Cooking Time: 20 Minutes

Servings: 2

Ingredients

4 fresh Nectarines sliced,

1 tablespoon honey

½ tablespoon coconut flour

1 tablespoon corn-starch

½ teaspoon lemon juice

1/2 cup Water

For the Topping

½ cup coconut flour

1 tablespoon honey

½ teaspoon baking powder

¼ teaspoon salt

2 tablespoon butter

¼ cup buttermilk

Instructions

Combine Nectarines, honey, coconut flour, corn-starch, lemon juice. Pour ½ cup water in the bottom of the Instant Pot, turn it on to sauté, and boil the water. Add the Nectarines and let it cook.

In the meantime, for the topping, mix the coconut flour, honey, baking powder, and salt together. Cut in the butter with a pastry cutter until pea size. Stir in the buttermilk.

Drop spoonful of the topping onto the Nectarines mixture, close the lid, select manual pressure high and set the time for 20 minutes. Natural pressure release and serve. Best served with vanilla ice cream.

Nutrition:

Calories 220, Total Fat 7.7g, Saturated Fat 5g, Cholesterol 16mg , Sodium 210mg, Total Carbohydrate 34.6g, Dietary Fiber 8.7g, Total Sugars 17.2g, Protein 3.8g

300. Hazelnuts Corn Syrup Mousse

Preparation Time: 15 Minutes

Cooking Time: 25 Minutes

Servings: 2

Ingredients

½ tablespoon butter melted

1 egg

½ cup heavy cream

¼ cup corn syrup

1 cup hazelnuts

Chocolate Ganache Topping optional

Instructions

Using a paper towel, coat the inside of a spring form cake pan or oven proof casserole pan with coconut oil.

Line the bottom and sides of the pan with parchment paper and set aside.

Put the egg, heavy cream, and corn syrup into a blender and mix, scraping down the sides as needed, until completely smooth. Pour the mixture into the pan.

Pour 1 cup of water into the Instant Pot and place the trivet inside. Place the pan on top of the trivet and close the lid tightly.

Press Manual and adjust time to 25 minutes pressure cooking. When the timer ends, let pressure naturally release.

Open the lid and carefully lift out the trivet and place the pan on a cooling rack for 30-45 minutes.

When cooled, invert the pan onto a platter, carefully lift out the parchment paper from the side.

Invert it again onto another platter, loosely cover and refrigerate overnight.

If you are using chocolate ganache topping, you can make it before serving, let it cool a little and cover the Hazelnuts Mousse and serve immediately.

Nutrition:

Calories 479, Total Fat 36.1g, Saturated Fat 9.3g, Cholesterol 123mg , Sodium 43mg, Total Carbohydrate 36.7g, Dietary Fiber 3.6g , Total Sugars 12g, Protein 9g

301. Coconut Brownies

Preparation Time: 15 Minutes

Cooking Time: 25 Minutes

Servings: 2

Ingredients

½ cup coconut flour

2 tablespoons honey

½ cup butter

¼ cup raw cacao powder

1 egg

1/8 teaspoon fine sea salt

¼ teaspoon baking soda

¼ teaspoon pure vanilla extract

¼ cup dark chocolate chips

Instructions

Line a 7-inch round pan with parchment paper. In a large bowl, combine the coconut flour, butter, honey, cacao powder, egg, salt, baking soda, and vanilla extract and stir well to create a thick batter.

Transfer the batter to the prepared pan and use your hands to press it evenly into the pan. Sprinkle with the chocolate chips and gently press them into the batter.

Pour 1 cup water into the Instant Pot and arrange the handled trivet on the bottom. Place the pan on top of the trivet and cover it with an upside-down plate or another piece of parchment to protect the brownies from condensation.

Secure the lid and move the steam release valve to Sealing. Select Manual/Pressure Cook to cook on high pressure for 15 minutes. When the cooking cycle is complete, let the pressure naturally release for 10 minutes, then move the steam release valve to Venting to release any remaining pressure. When the floating valve drops, remove the lid.

Let the brownies cool completely in the pan before cutting and serving.

Nutrition:

Calories 294, Total Fat 26.4g, Saturated Fat 16.4g, Cholesterol 102mg , Sodium 321mg, Total Carbohydrate 14.8g, Dietary Fiber 0.7g, Total Sugars 12.9g, Protein 2.4g

302. Dates and Almond Halwa

Preparation Time: 10 Minutes

Cooking Time: 20 Minutes

Servings: 2

Ingredients

1 cup dates, dried, stemmed and coarsely chopped

½ cup water

½ cup almonds finely chopped

½ cup shelled pine nuts finely chopped

1 tablespoon coconut oil

¼ teaspoon cardamom ground

Instructions

Combine the dates and water in the Instant Pot.

Secure the lid and set the Pressure Release to Sealing. Select the Pressure Cook or Manual setting and set the cooking time for 5 minutes at high pressure.

Perform a quick release by moving the Pressure Release to Venting. Open the pot and coarsely mash the dates with a potato masher or wooden spatula.

Add the almonds, pine nuts, coconut oil, and cardamom and stir together. Press the Cancel button to reset the cooking program, then select the low Sauté setting and cook the Halwa, stirring frequently, until it thickens to a pudding-like consistency, about 10 minutes. Press the Cancel button to turn off the Instant Pot.

Spoon the Halwa into bowls and serve.

Nutrition:

Calories 310, Total Fat 7.2g, Saturated Fat 5.9g, Cholesterol 0mg , Sodium 4mg, Total Carbohydrate 66.8g, Dietary Fiber 7.1g, Total Sugars 56.4g, Protein 2.2g

303. Fudge Pine nuts Brownies

Preparation Time: 10 Minutes

Cooking Time: 35 Minutes

Servings: 2

Ingredients

½ cup oats flour

1/8 teaspoon baking powder

1/8 teaspoon salt

1 cup coconut sugar

½ cup coconut oil, softened

2 eggs

2 cups squares unsweetened baking chocolate, melted

½ teaspoon vanilla extract

1 cup coarsely chopped Pine nuts

Instructions

Grease an 8x8-inch square pan.

Sift oats flour, baking powder, and salt together in a bowl.

Beat coconut sugar and coconut oil together in a large bowl with an electric mixer until light and fluffy. Beat in eggs until smooth batter forms; beat in chocolate and vanilla extract. Stir oats flour mixture in just until incorporated; fold in pine nuts. Spread batter into prepared square pan.

Pour 1 cup water into the Instant Pot and arrange the handled trivet on the bottom. Place the pan on top of the trivet and cover it with an upside-down plate or another piece of parchment to protect the brownies from condensation.

Secure the lid and move the steam release valve to Sealing. Select Manual/Pressure Cook to cook on high pressure for 30 minutes. When the cooking cycle is complete, let the pressure naturally release for 10 minutes, then move the steam release valve to Venting to release any remaining pressure. When the floating valve drops, remove the lid.

Let the brownies cool completely in the pan before cutting and serving.

Nutrition:

Calories334, Total Fat 29.5g, Saturated Fat 12.6g, Cholesterol 63mg, Sodium 134mg, Total Carbohydrate 14.5g, Dietary Fiber 0.6g , Total Sugars 12.9g, Protein 4.7g

304. Nectarine and Sunflower seed Rice Pudding

Preparation Time: 05 Minutes

Cooking Time: 10 Minutes

Servings: 2

Ingredients

¼ cup short-grain white rice well rinsed and drained

2 cups coconut milk

1 tablespoon honey

1 pinch salt

1 large egg beaten, at room temperature

½ tablespoon sunflower seed

¼ teaspoon vanilla extract

1 small Nectarine peeled and diced

Instructions

Combine the rice, coconut milk, honey, and salt in your Instant Pot. Whisk together and secure the lid.

Cook at high pressure for 10 minutes and use a natural release.

Whisk the cooked rice and milk mixture well. Temper the eggs by slowly adding 1 cup of the hot milky rice to the egg while whisking constantly. Add that mixture to the Instant Pot slowly, whisking the whole time.

Turn on the Sauté function. Whisk until the mixture is simmering and starting to thicken up. Turn off the Sauté function.

Add the sunflower seed and vanilla and mix well.

Allow the rice pudding to cool. It will thicken greatly as it sits. Serve warm or cold topped with fresh nectarine.

Nutrition:

Calories 340, Total Fat 30.2g, Saturated Fat 25.8g, Cholesterol 47mg, Sodium 75mg, Total Carbohydrate 17.4g, Dietary Fiber 3.3g, Total Sugars 11.3g, Protein 5g

305. Chocolate-Almond Butter Cups

Preparation Time: 15 Minutes

Cooking Time: 05 Minutes

Servings: 2

Ingredients

¼ cup butter

¼ cup natural almond butter

1 tablespoon coconut cream

1 teaspoon cocoa powder

1 teaspoon maple syrup

¼ teaspoon vanilla extract

¼ teaspoon salt

½ cup chopped roasted salted almonds

Instructions

Select Sauté in Instant pot and Melt butter. Stir in almond butter until smooth. Whisk in coconut cream, cocoa powder, honey, vanilla extract, and salt.

Close the lid of Instant pot. Cook at high pressure for 03 minutes and use a natural release.

Pour chocolate-almond butter mixture into silicone muffin molds. Sprinkle almonds evenly on top. Place molds on a baking sheet.

Freeze chocolate-peanut butter mixture until firm, at least 1 hour. Unmould chocolate-almonds cups and transfer to a resalable plastic bag or airtight container.

Nutrition:

Calories116, Total Fat 12.5g, Saturated Fat 8.1g, Cholesterol 31mg, Sodium 230mg, Total Carbohydrate 1.6g, Dietary Fiber 0.2g, Total Sugars 1.2g, Protein 0.3g

306. Plum Skillet Cake

Preparation Time: 15 Minutes

Cooking Time: 05 Minutes

Servings: 2

Ingredients

2½ tablespoon coconut oil

½ cup almond flour

¼ teaspoon salt

¼ teaspoon baking powder

1/8 teaspoon baking soda

2 tablespoon honey

1 large egg

½ cup low-fat buttermilk

2 medium ripe plums, pitted and thinly sliced

2 tablespoons coconut sugar

Instructions

Butter an 8-inch cast iron or oven-proof skillet. Dust with flour, tapping out any excess.

Whisk together almond flour, salt, baking powder, and baking soda in a medium bowl.

Combine coconut oil and honey in a large bowl; beat with an electric mixer on medium speed until pale and fluffy. Beat in egg. Add flour mixture in 3 batches, alternating with buttermilk, beating batter briefly after each addition.

Pour batter into the prepared skillet and smooth the top with an offset spatula. Fan plum slices on top of batter, and sprinkle with remaining coconut sugar.

Pour 1 cup water into the Instant Pot and arrange the handled trivet on the bottom. Place the pan on top of the trivet and cover it with an upside-down plate or another piece of parchment to protect the brownies from condensation.

Secure the lid and move the steam release valve to Sealing. Select Manual/Pressure Cook to cook on high pressure for 45 minutes. When the cooking cycle is complete, let the pressure naturally release for 10 minutes, then move the steam release valve to Venting to release any remaining pressure. When the floating valve drops, remove the lid.

Let cool slightly before serving.

Nutrition:

Calories 385, Total Fat 37.3g, Saturated Fat 31.4g, Cholesterol 48mg, Sodium 236mg, Total Carbohydrate 14.4g, Dietary Fiber 0.5g , Total Sugars 13.7g, Protein 2.9g

307. Yellow Squash Brownies

Preparation Time: 15 Minutes

Cooking Time: 30 Minutes

Servings: 2

Ingredients

1 tablespoons coconut oil

½ tablespoons honey

½ teaspoon vanilla extract

1 cup coconut flour

½ tablespoon unsweetened cocoa powder

½ teaspoon baking soda

1/8 teaspoon salt

1 cup shredded yellow squash

¼ cup chopped walnuts

Instructions

Grease and flour a 9x13 inch baking pan.

In a large bowl, mix together the coconut oil, honey and 2 teaspoons vanilla until well blended. Combine the coconut flour, cocoa, baking soda and salt; stir into the honey mixture. Fold in the yellow squash and walnuts. Spread evenly into the prepared pan.

Pour 1 cup water into the Instant Pot and arrange the handled trivet on the bottom. Place the pan on top of the trivet and cover it with an upside-down plate or another piece of parchment to protect the brownies from condensation.

Secure the lid and move the steam release valve to Sealing. Select Manual/Pressure Cook to cook on high pressure for 45 minutes. When the cooking cycle is complete, let the pressure naturally release for 10 minutes, then move the steam release valve to Venting to release any remaining pressure. When the floating valve drops, remove the lid.

Let cool slightly before serving.

Nutrition:

Calories108, Total Fat 8.7g, Saturated Fat 3.8g, Cholesterol 0mg , Sodium 243mg, Total Carbohydrate 6.3g, Dietary Fiber 2.3g, Total Sugars 3.1g, Protein 2.9g

308. Apple Pie Quinoa Pudding

Preparation Time: 05 Minutes

Cooking Time: 10 Minutes

Servings: 2

Ingredients

2 cups quinoa

2 cups apples finely chopped

1 cup soy milk

½ tablespoon cinnamon powder

½ tablespoon Vanilla free

1/8 teaspoon ground cardamom

½ cup golden dates

Instructions

Place all Ingredients in the Instant Pot.

Cook on manual at high pressure for 10 minutes. When time is up, quick release the pressure.

Serve and enjoy! This is delicious served hot, warm or cold.

Nutrition:

Calories 239, Total Fat 2.7g, Saturated Fat 0.3g, Cholesterol 0mg , Sodium 34mg, Total Carbohydrate 50.5g, Dietary Fiber 6.8g, Total Sugars 28.4g, Protein 5.9g

309. Dulbecco,

Preparation Time: 05 Minutes

Cooking Time: 45 Minutes

Servings: 2

Ingredients

½ cup sweetened condensed milk

1 cup water

½ teaspoon sea salt

Chopped walnuts for topping

Chopped chocolate

Instructions

Pour the water into the Instant pot, and place the trivet inside. Place the ramekins on the trivet, stacking them if needed. Lock the lid into place. Select Pressure Cook or Manual, and adjust the pressure to High and the time to 45 minutes. Make sure the steam release knob is in the sealed position.

After cooking, naturally release the pressure. Unlock and remove the lid. Carefully remove the ramekins. Remove the foil, and sprinkle with the sea salt. Let cool for 30 minutes before topping with chopped walnuts and chocolate, if desired, and serving.

Nutrition:

Calories 288, Total Fat 10g, Saturated Fat 5.1g , Cholesterol 27mg, Sodium 572mg, Total Carbohydrate 44.1g, Dietary Fiber 0.4g, Total Sugars 43.5g, Protein 7.3g

310. Baked Peaches

Preparation Time: 10 Minutes

Cooking Time: 15 Minutes

Servings: 2

Ingredients

1/8 cup apricots

1/8 cup dates chopped

1/8 cup walnuts chopped

1 teaspoon nutmeg

1 tablespoon honey

4 small peaches

2 tablespoons coconut oil

1 cup Water

Instructions

In a small bowl, mix apricots, dates, walnuts, nutmeg and honey.

Using a melon baller or paring knife, remove the peaches cores, leaving the bottom 1/2 inch of the peaches intact.

Fill apples with filling mixture and top each with a thin slice of butter.

Pour 2/3 cup water in the Instant Pot and arrange the apples in the bottom of the pot. Add any extra butter to the cooking water.

Secure the lid, making sure the vent is closed.

Using the display panel select the MANUAL or PRESSURE COOK function*. Use the + /- keys and program the Instant Pot for 3 minutes.

When the time is up, let the pressure naturally release for 5 minutes, then quick-release the remaining pressure.

Serve warm.

Nutrition:

Calories278, Total Fat 14.9g, Saturated Fat 12.1g, Cholesterol 0mg, Sodium 4mg, Total Carbohydrate 38.3g, Dietary Fiber 5g , Total Sugars 37.8g, Protein 3g

311. Zucchini Bars

Preparation Time: 10 minutes

Cooking time: 15 minutes

Servings: 10

Ingredients:

1 zucchini, shredded

1 cup almond flour

¼ cup coconut butter

½ teaspoon baking powder

1 teaspoon lemon juice

1/3 cup Erythritol

1 teaspoon vanilla extract

Directions:

In the mixing bowl combine together shredded zucchini, almond flour, baking powder, lemon juice, and Erythritol.

Stir gently and add coconut butter and vanilla extract.

Mix up the mixture with the help of the spoon and place it in the lined with the parchment baking tray.

Flatten the mixture and cook it on 365F for 15 minutes.

After this, remove the zucchini dessert from the oven and cut it into the bars with the help of a pizza knife.

Nutrition: calories 58, fat 5, fiber 2.5, carbs 10.4, protein 1.2

312. Coconut Cookies

Preparation Time: 10 minutes

Cooking time: 10 minutes

Servings: 12

Ingredients:

1 cup coconut flour

½ cup coconut shred

2 egg whites

3 tablespoon Erythritol

1 tablespoon coconut oil

Directions:

 Whisk the eggs whites until you get soft peaks.

 Combine together whisked egg whites, coconut shred, coconut flour, and Erythritol.

 Stir gently and add coconut oil.

 Mix up the mixture until homogenous.

 Make the small size cooked from the coconut mixture and press them gently.

 Line the baking tray with the baking paper.

 Place the cookies on the tray and cook them at 365F for 10 minutes. Check the cookies after 5 minutes of cooking.

 When the cookies are cooked – chill them till the room temperature and store in the closed glass jar.

Nutrition: calories 75, fat 4.4, fiber 4.4, carbs 11.3, protein 2.2

313. Red Velvet Muffins

Preparation Time: 10 minutes

Cooking time: 10 minutes

Servings: 6

Ingredients:

3 tablespoon almond butter

¼ cup almond milk

1 teaspoon vanilla extract

½ teaspoon baking powder

1 cup almond flour

1 teaspoon red food coloring

Directions:

Melt the almond butter and combine it together with the vanilla extract and food coloring.

When the mixture is smooth – add baking powder, almond milk, and almond flour.

Make the homogenous batter.

Preheat the oven to 360F.

Fill ½ part of every muffin mold with the red batter.

Transfer the molds in the oven and cook for 10 minutes.

Check the muffins with the help of the toothpick and cook them for 2-3 minutes more if need.

Nutrition: calories 186, fat 15.8, fiber 3, carbs 6.3, protein 5.9

314.   Gingerbread Muffins

Preparation Time: 8 minutes

Cooking time: 11 minutes

Servings: 10

Ingredients:

1 cup coconut flour

1 cup almond flour

1/2 cup heavy cream

4 tablespoon Erythritol

1 teaspoon vanilla extract

1 teaspoon ground ginger

1/2 teaspoon ground cinnamon

1/2 teaspoon ground cloves

Directions:

Mix up together all the ingredients in the mixing bowl.

Use the hand mixer to make the mixture smooth and homogenous.

After this, fill ½ part of every muffin mold with the smooth batter.

Cook the muffins at 365F for 11 minutes.

When the time is over – chill the muffins till the room temperature.

Nutrition: calories 45, fat 3.9, fiber 0.9, carbs 7.9, protein 1

DAY	BREAKFAST	MAINS	SNACK/DESSERT
1.	Breakfast Pudding - Apple Crumble	Vegan Sausage Collard Rolls	Vanilla Pudding
2.	Broccoli & Tofu Stuffed Pita Pockets	Cauliflower Stew	Quick Cherry Crisp
3.	Eggless Garlic Bread Rolls	Seitan Cauliflower Bowl	Chocolate Chip Cheesecake
4.	Onion Stuffed Flatbread	Cheesy Mushroom in Omelet	Peanut Butter Fudge
5.	Cranberry & Almond Biscotti	Tomato Cream	Banana-Oatmeal Cake
6.	Corn Muffins	Cajun Tofu in Mushrooms	Fresh Apple Cake
7.	Quinoa & Flax Muffins	Braised Seitan with Kelp Noodles	Apple Banana Cupcakes
8.	Sweet Potato Cornbread	Stewed Tofu with Walnut Cauliflower Grits	Banana Chocolate Chip Cake
9.	Almond & Pomegranate Scones	Tempeh Zucchini Mug Melt	Blueberry Buttermilk Coffeecake
10.	Rosemary & Blueberry Scones	Fennel and Rice	Prunes Cake

No.			
11.	Cinnamon Flavored Blueberry Coffee Cake	Kale and Mushroom Pierogis	Butternut squash -Almond Cookies
12.	Apple Butter Sauce	Tempeh Coconut Curry Bake	Nectarine and Sunflower seed Rice Pudding
13.	No-Knead Bread	Avocado Coconut Pie	Gingerbread Muffins
14.	Oat and whole wheat bread	Spicy Cheese with Tofu Balls	Red Velvet Muffins
15.	Hot Chocolate Steel-Cut Oatmeal	Tempeh with Garlic Asparagus	Zucchini Bars
16.	Apple Cinnamon Oatmeal	Pimiento Tofu balls	Coconut Cookies
17.	Blueberry Oatmeal Waffles	Baked Mushrooms with Creamy Brussels Sprouts	Baked Peaches
18.	Pumpkin Granola	Mushroom Curry Pie	Apple Pie Quinoa Pudding
19.	Herb Bread	Seitan Tex-Mex Casserole	Yellow Squash Brownies
20.	Grain Porridge	Tofu Loco Moco	Plum Skillet Cake
21.	Pecan Buns	Tempeh Mushroom Omelet	Chocolate-Almond Butter Cups

Conclusion

I hope that you and your loved ones will enjoy dining on this collection of wonderfully healthy vegetarian keto meals, snacks, and desserts. I can say that a meal tastes so much better when I know that it is a healthy choice in foods. However, it is even more enjoyable when it is a healthy meal that tastes great—this is what I would call a win-win! I hope that you will find this collection of recipes a big win for you—hopefully becoming some of your favorite dishes!